MW00510307

Keto Diet Cookbook for Beginners

Juicy Keto Meals Guaranteed To Raise Your Energy Levels And Improve Your Mood

By

Casey Black

Table of Contents

Keto Dessert & Chaffle Cookbook 2021 with Pictures

Intermittent Fasting for Women Over 60

The Healthy Keto Meal Prep Cookbook with Pictures

Intermittent Fasting for Women

Keto diet Cookbook

Recipes **408**

Keto Dessert & Chaffle Cookbook 2021 with Pictures

Quick and Easy, Sugar-Low Bombs, Chaffle and Cakes Recipes to Shed Weight, Boost Your Mood and Live Ketogenic lifestyle

By

Casey Black

Table of Contents

Introduction

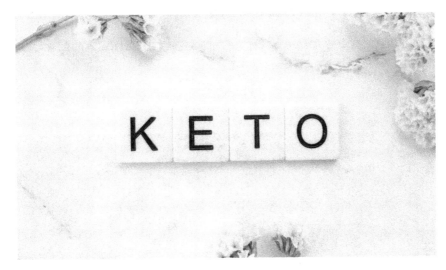

The ketogenic diet or Keto is a low-carbohydrate, mild protein, high-fat diet that will help you lose fat more efficiently. It has several advantages for weight reduction, wellbeing, and efficiency, so a rising number of healthcare professionals & practitioners recommend it.

Fat as a form of nutrition

For nutrition, the body uses three fuel sources: carbohydrates, fats and proteins. Carbohydrates convert into blood sugar or glucose in the bloodstream and are the primary fuel source for the body. If carbohydrates are not accessible, your body then depends on fat as an energy source. Protein is the primary building block of muscles and tissues. Protein could also be processed into glucose in a pinch and utilized for energy.

The keto diet encourages your body to utilize fat as the primary source of nutrition instead of carbohydrates, a ketosis mechanism. You consume too little carbs on the keto diet that the body cannot depend on glucose for nutrition. And your body turns to utilize fat for energy rather than carbs, as keto foods are filled with fat. A major part of the calories, almost 70 to 80% come from fat, consuming 15 to 20% of calories from protein and barely 5% calories from carbohydrates (that makes for about 20 to 30 grams of carbohydrates per day, depending on the weight and height of a person).

Meal options in regular diets

To conquer the weight reduction fight, it becomes tough to continue the dieting combat for a long period. Many people revert to the previous eating patterns after only a few weeks when confronted with the difficulty and limited food ranges of many diets, especially vegan, low-fat and low-calorie diets. For starters, the ketogenic diet is incredibly beneficial for weight reduction, but following specific food choices can be overwhelming. Only after three weeks can you begin noticing significant effects; however, the complications and inconvenience of transitioning to an effective ketogenic diet may deter you from keeping to the program long enough to reap the benefits.

Thankfully, to render your keto diet ever more efficient, successful and simple to use, you will build an array of foods, preparing strategies, tips and suggestions. One hidden tool can be used from the diet's outset, without much details of the keto diet, which is continued even after achieving the weight loss target.

That hidden preferred weapon is the "Fat Bomb."

The Fat Bomb

The fat bombs in the keto diet play a major role in motivation for the dieters. Indulging in a high fat dessert gives you a stress-free environment to continue your diet. These fat bombs provide the correct amounts of fat, carbohydrates, and protein resulting in weight reduction while supplying the user with sustained energy. They do this by supplementing your diet with chemicals that hold your body in a fat-burning state, even after you have had a fulfilling meal.

The Keto diet aims to rely on foods that are high in fat and low in carbs. By modifying what the body utilizes as food, it helps facilitate weight reduction. Carbohydrates, like those present in sugars and bread, are usually transformed into energy. If the body cannot have enough nutrients, the body begins to burn fat as a substitute for energy.

Your liver converts the fat into ketones, which are a form of acid. Getting a certain amount of ketones in your body will lead you to a biochemical condition known as ketosis. Your body can burn stored fat for fuel; thus, you will losing weight when you go through ketosis.

To reach a ketosis condition, it takes between one to ten days of consuming a low-carb, high-fat diet; to sustain the fat-burning cycle of ketosis, you have to continue consuming the keto diet. Eating fatty foods will help you more easily get into ketosis and sustain it for longer periods.

Fat bombs are 90% fat, making them the ideal keto addition for beginners and lifetime keto adherents. They hold you in a ketosis state and can provide health advantages unlike many other high protein foods; you can snack on fat bombs or have them as dinners or as have as a side dish too. They are simple to produce and are available in a range of varieties, from sweet to savory.

Can Fat Bombs Be Healthy?

Ketogenic fat bombs are fueled by two major ingredients: high-fat dairy and coconut oil. Both of these components have several powerful health advantages. Coconut produces a form of fat known as MCTs (medium-chain triglycerides), which gives the body additional ketones that can be readily consumed and used to sustain ketosis.

There are distinct health advantages of consuming high-fat dairy fat bombs. High-fat dairy products produce fatty acids known as CLA (conjugated linoleic acid), minerals and vitamins. Data indicates that CLA plays a significant role in the body's breakdown of fat and may lower cardiac attack and stroke risk.

Eating high-fat dairy meals prior to bedtime may help burn fat when still sleeping. Fat burned while you sleep the body with an energy that does not need to metabolize stress hormones or depend on sugar.

Keto Diet and Mood

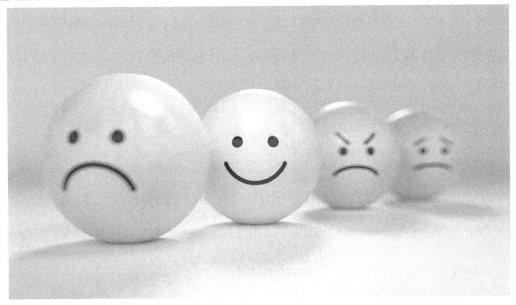

There are various comments from individuals on a keto diet that probably indicate the association between the keto diet and mood changes. Various hypotheses connect the keto diet to mood regulation, even if only partly.

The explanation of why the keto diet aids in accelerated weight reduction and reversal of multiple chronic weight-related problems lead people to come out of the despair of "I am not healthy." As a consequence of the results themselves, most people report a positive attitude by adopting a keto diet. But is that important? What makes a difference is that it has a positive and long-lasting effect. Some research also shows that a ketogenic diet may help combat depression since it provides anti-inflammatory benefits. Inflammations are associated with, at least certain, forms of depression. A few of the advantages are provided below that create the relationship between the keto diet and mood. A keto diet:

1. Helps regulate energy highs and lows.

Ketones offer an immediate energy supply for your brain since they are metabolized quicker than glucose. Ketones give a long-lasting, more accurate and reliable energy supply, and when your body understands it can access your fat reserves for food as well, the brain does not worry.

2. Neurogenesis improvement

Dietary consumption is a crucial element in assessing neurogenesis. A reduced degree of neurogenesis is correlated with multiple depressive illnesses. On the other side, a higher rate increases emotional endurance.

3. Reduces and Brings Down Inflammation

The Keto Diet provides healthy nutritional options, so you avoid consuming inflammatory and refined products. Consuming anti-inflammatory food can have a direct impact on the attitude. If you eat nutritious food high in protein, healthy fats and low-carb vegetables, it reduces inflammation.

4. Feeds the brain.

The good fat you consume on Keto fuels your brain and stabilizes your mood. As your brain is composed of 60% fat, it requires an excess of healthy fats to function properly.

So go ahead and try these easy to make lo carb hi fat desserts and lose weight deliciously!

Chapter 1- Low Carb Desserts

1. 10 Minutes Chocolate Mousse

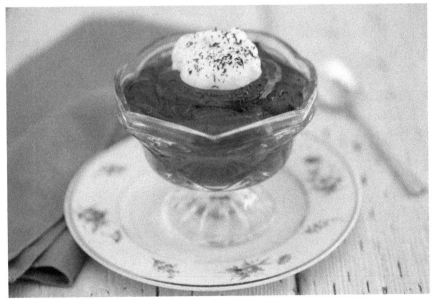

Prep. Time: 10 minutes

Servings: 4

The serving size is ½ cup

Nutrition as per serving:

218 kcal / 23g fat / 5g carbs / 2g fiber / 2g protein = 3g net carbs

Ingredients

- Powdered sweetener 1/4 cup

- Cocoa powder, unsweetened, sifted 1/4 cup

- Vanilla extract 1tsp.

- Heavy whipping cream 1 cup

- Kosher salt 1/4tsp.

Directions

With an electric beater, beat the cream to form stiff peaks. Put in the sweetener, cocoa powder, salt, vanilla and whisk till all ingredients are well combined.

2. The Best Keto Cheesecake

Prep. Time: 20 minutes

Cook Time: 50 minutes

Setting Time: 8 hours

Servings: 12

The serving size is 1 slice

Nutrition as per serving:

600kcal / 54g fat / 7g carbs / 2g fiber / 14g protein = 5 g net carbs

Ingredients

Layer of crust

- Powdered sweetener 1/4 cup

- Almond flour 1 1/2 cups

- Butter melted 6 tbsp.

- Cinnamon 1tsp.

Filling

- Cream cheese, full fat, room temperature (8 oz.)

- Powdered Sweetener 2 Cups

- Eggs at room temperature 5 Large

- Sour cream at room temperature 8 Oz.

- Vanilla extract 1 Tbsp.

Directions

1. Heat the oven to 325F.

2. Arrange the rack in the center of the oven. Mix dry ingredients for the crust in a medium mixing bowl. Mix in the butter. Transfer the crust mixture into a springform pan (10-inch x 4- inch), and using your fingers, press halfway up and around the sides. Then press the mixture with a flat bottom cup into the pan. Chill the crust for about 20 minutes.

3. Beat the cream cheese (at room temperature) in a large mixing container, with an electric beater or a

4. Hand mixer until fluffy and light.

5. If using a stand mixer, attach the paddle accessory.

6. Add in about 1/3rd of sweetener at a time and beat well.

7. Add in one egg at a time beating until well incorporated.

8. Lastly, add in the sour cream, vanilla and mix until just combined.

9. Pour this cheesecake mixture onto the crust and smooth out the top. Place in the heated oven and examine after 50 minutes. The center should not jiggle, and the top should not be glossy anymore.

10. Turn the oven off and open the door slightly, leaving the cheesecake inside for about 30 minutes.

11. Take out the cheesecake and run a knife between the pan and the cheesecake (this is to unstick the cake but don't remove the springform yet). Leave for 1 hour.

12. Chill for at least 8 hrs. loosely covered with plastic wrap.

13. Take off the sides of the springform pan, decorate & serve.

Note: all the ingredients to make the cheesecake should be at room temperature. Anything refrigerated must be left out for at least 4 hrs.

3. Butter Pralines

Prep. Time: 5 minutes

Cook Time: 11 minutes

Chilling Time: 1 hour

Servings: 10

The serving size is 2 Butter Pralines

Nutrition as per serving:

338kcal / 36g fat / 3g carbs / 2g fiber / 2g protein = 1g net carbs

Ingredients

• Salted butter 2 Sticks

• Heavy Cream 2/3 Cup

• Granular Sweetener 2/3 Cup

- Xanthan gum ½ tsp.

- Chopped pecans 2 Cups

- Sea salt

Directions

1. Line parchment paper on a cookie sheet with or apply a silicone baking mat on it.

2. In a saucepan, brown the butter on medium-high heat, stirring regularly, for just about 5 minutes.

3. Add in the sweetener, heavy cream and xanthan gum. Stir and take off the heat.

4. Add in the nuts and chill to firm up, occasionally stirring, for about 1 hour. The mixture will become very thick. Shape into ten cookie forms and place on the lined baking sheet, and sprinkle with the sea salt, if preferred. Let chill until hardened.

5. Keep in a sealed container, keep refrigerated until serving.

4. Homemade Healthy Twix Bars

Prep. Time: 5 minutes

Cook Time: 20 minutes

Servings: 18 Bars

The serving size is 1 Bar

Nutrition as per serving:

111kcal / 7g fat / 8g carbs / 5g fiber / 4g protein = 3g net carbs

Ingredients

For the cookie layer

- Coconut flour 3/4 cup

- Almond flour 1 cup

- Keto maple syrup 1/4 cup

- Sweetener, granulated 1/2 cup

- Flourless keto cookies 1/4 cup

- Almond milk 1/2 cup

For the gooey caramel

- Cashew butter (or any seed or nut butter) 1 cup

- Sticky sweetener of choice 1 cup

- Coconut oil 1 cup

- For the chocolate coating

- Chocolate chips 2 cups

Directions

1. Line parchment paper in a loaf pan or square pan and set aside.

2. In a big mixing bowl, put in almond flour, coconut flour, and then granulated. Combine very well. Mix in the keto syrup and stir to make it into a thick dough.

3. Add the crushed keto cookies and also add a tbsp. of milk to keep it a thick batter. If the batter stays too thick, keep adding milk by tablespoon. Once desired consistency is achieved, shift the batter to the prepared pan and smooth it out. Chill.

4. Combine the cashew butter, coconut oil and syrup on the stovetop or a microwave-safe dish and heat until mixed. Beat very well to make sure the coconut oil is completely mixed. Drizzle the caramel over the prepared cookie layer and shift to the freezer.

5. When the bars are hard, take out of the pan and slice into 18 bars. Once more, put it back in the freezer.

6. Liquefy the chocolate chips by heat. Using two forks, dip each Twix bar into the melted chocolate till evenly covered. Cover all the bars with chocolate. Chill until firm.

5. Best Chocolate Chip cookie

Prep. Time: 5 minutes

Cook Time: 20 minutes

Servings: 15 Cookies

The serving size is 1 Cookie

Nutrition as per serving:

98kcal / 6g fat / 12g carbs / 5g fiber / 5g protein = 7g net carbs

Ingredients

- Almond flour blanched 2 cups
- Baking powder 1 tsp
- Cornstarch 1/4 cup
- Coconut oil 2 tbsp.
- Sticky sweetener, keto-friendly 6 tbsp.
- Almond extract 1 tsp
- Coconut milk, unsweetened 1/4 cup
- Chocolate chips 1/2 cup

Directions

1. Heat oven up to 350F/175C. Line parchment paper on a large cookie tray and put it aside.

2. Place all the dry ingredients in a big mixing bowl, and combine well.

3. Melt the keto-friendly-sticky sweetener, almond extract and coconut oil in a microwave-safe proof or stovetop. Then mix it into the dry mixture, adding milk to combine very well. Stir through your chocolate chips.

4. Form small balls with slightly wet hands from the cookie dough. Set the balls up on the lined cookie tray. Then form them into cookies by pressing them with a fork. Bake for 12 to 15 minutes till they brown.

5. Take out from the oven, allowing to cool on the tray completely.

6. White Chocolate Dairy Free Peanut Butter Cups

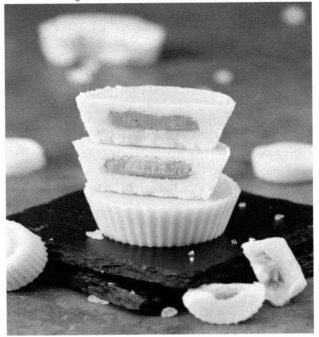

Prep. Time: 5 minutes

Cook Time: 5 minutes

Servings: 40

The serving size is 1 cup

Nutrition as per serving:

117kcal / 6g fat / 14g carbs / 10g fiber / 3g protein = 4g net carbs

Ingredients

- White Chocolate Bar, Sugar-free, coarsely chopped 4 cups

- Peanut butter, smooth (or sunflower seed butter) 1 cup

- Coconut flour 2 tbsp.

- Unsweetened coconut milk 2 tbsp.+ more if needed

Directions

1. Line muffin liners in a standard muffin tin of 12 cups or mini muffin tin of 20 cups and put aside.

2. Removing ½ a cup of your white chocolate, melt the remaining 3 1/2 cups on the stovetop or in a microwave-safe dish, till silky and smooth. Quickly, pour the melted white chocolate equally amongst the prepared muffin cups, scrape down the sides to remove all. Once done, chill

3. Meanwhile, start making the peanut butter filling. Mix the flour and peanut butter well. Adding a tsp. of milk at a time brings to the desired texture.

4. Take the hardened white chocolate cups, then equally pour the peanut butter filling among all of them. After all, is used up, take white chocolate that was kept aside and melt them. Then pour it on each of the cups to cover fully. Chill until firm.

7. Chocolate Crunch Bars

Prep. Time: 5 minutes

Cook Time: 5 minutes

Servings: 20 servings

The serving size is 1 Bar

Nutrition as per serving:

155kcal / 12g fat / 4g carbs / 2g fiber / 7g protein = 2g net carbs

Ingredients

• Chocolate chips (stevia sweetened), 1 1/2 cups

• Almond butter (or any seed or nut butter) 1 cup

- Sticky sweetener (swerve sweetened or monk fruit syrup) 1/2 cup

- Coconut oil 1/4 cup

- Seeds and nuts (like almonds, pepitas, cashews, etc.) 3 cups

Directions

1. Line parchment paper on a baking dish of 8 x 8-inch and put it aside.

2. Combine the keto-friendly chocolate chips, coconut oil, almond butter and sticky sweetener and melt on a stovetop or a microwave-safe dish until combined.

3. Include nuts and seeds and combine until fully mixed. Pour this mixture into the parchment-lined baking dish smoothing it out with a spatula. Chill until firm.

Notes

Keep refrigerated

8. Easy Peanut Butter Cups

Prep. Time: 10minutes

Cook Time: 5minutes

Servings: 12

The serving size is 1 piece

Nutrition as per serving:

187kcal / 18g fat / 14g carbs / 11g fiber / 3g protein = 3g net carbs

Ingredients

Chocolate layers

- Dark chocolate(not bakers chocolate), Sugar-free, 10 oz. Divided
- Coconut oil 5 tbsp. (divided)
- Vanilla extracts 1/2 tsp. (divided) optional

Peanut butter layer

- Creamy Peanut butter 3 1/2 tbsp.

- Coconut oil 2 tsp.

- Powdered Erythritol (or to taste) 4 tsp.

- Peanut flour 1 1/2 tsp.

- Vanilla extracts 1/8 tsp. Optional

- Sea salt 1 pinch (or to taste) optional

Directions

1. Line parchment liners in a muffin pan

2. Prepare the chocolate layer on the stove, place a double boiler and heat half of the coconut oil and half of the chocolate, stirring regularly, until melted. (Alternatively use a microwave, heat for 20 seconds, stirring at intervals.). Add in half of the vanilla.

3. Fill each lined muffin cup with about 2 tsp. Of chocolate in each. Chill for around 10 minutes till the tops are firm.

4. Prepare the peanut butter filling: in a microwave or a double boiler, heat the coconut oil and peanut butter (similar to step 2). Mix in the peanut flour, powdered sweetener, sea salt and vanilla until smooth. Adjust salt and sweetener to taste if preferred.

5. Pour a tsp. Of the prepared peanut mixture into each cup with the chocolate layer. You don't want it to reach the edges. Chill for 10 minutes more till the tops are firm.

6. Now, prepare a chocolate layer for the top. Heat the leftover coconut oil and chocolate in a microwave or the double boiler (similar to step 2). Add in the vanilla.

7. Pour about 2 tsp of melted chocolate into each cup. It should cover the empty part and the peanut butter circles completely.

8. Again chill for at least 20 to 30 minutes, until completely solid. Keep in the refrigerator.

9. No-Bake Chocolate Coconut Bars

Prep. Time: 1 minute

Cook Time: 5 minutes

Servings: 12 bars

The serving size is 1 bar

Nutrition as per serving:

169 kcal / 17g fat / 5g carbs / 4g fiber / 2g protein = 1g net carbs

Ingredients

- Keto maple syrup 1/4 cup

- Coconut unsweetened, shredded 3 cups

- Coconut oil, melted 1 cup

- Lily's chocolate chips 1-2 cups

Directions

1. Line parchment paper in a large loaf pan or square pan and put aside.

2. Add all the ingredients to a large bowl and combine very well. Shift mixture to the prepared pan. Wet your hands lightly and press them into place. Chill for 30 minutes until firm. Cut into 12 bars.

3. Melt the sugar-free chocolate chips, and using two forks, dip each chilled bar into the melted chocolate and coat evenly. Evenly coat all the bars in the same way. Chill until chocolate solidifies.

4. Keep the Bars in a sealed container at room temperature. If you refrigerated or freeze them, thaw them completely before enjoying them.

10. Chocolate Peanut Butter Hearts

Prep. Time: 5 minutes

Cook Time: 5 minutes

Servings: 20 Hearts

The serving size is 1 Heart

Nutrition as per serving:

95kcal / 6g fat / 7g carbs / 5g fiber / 5g protein = 2g net carbs

Ingredients

- Smooth peanut butter 2 cups
- Sticky sweetener 3/4 cup
- Coconut flour 1 cup
- Chocolate chips of choice 1-2 cups

Directions

1. Line parchment paper on a large tray and put it aside.
2. Combine the keto-friendly sticky sweetener and peanut butter and melt on a stovetop or microwave-safe bowl until combined.
3. Include coconut flour and combine well. If the mixture is too thin, include more coconut flour. Leave for around 10 minutes to thicken.
4. Shape the peanut butter mixture into 18 to 20 small balls. Press each ball in. Then, using a heart-molded cookie cutter, shape the balls into hearts removing excess

peanut butter mixture from the sides. Assemble the hearts on the lined tray and chill.

5. Melt the keto-friendly chocolate chips. With two forks, coat the chocolate by dipping each heart into it. Repeat with all hearts. When done, chill until firm.

Notes

Keep in a sealed jar at room temperature for up to 2 weeks, or refrigerate for up to 2 months.

11. Magic Cookies

Prep. Time: 10 minutes

Cook Time: 15 minutes

Servings: 15 cookies

The serving size is 1 cookie

Nutrition as per serving:

130kcal / 13g fat / 2g carbs / 1g fiber / 2g protein = 1g net carbs

Ingredients

- Butter softened 3 tbsp.
- Coconut oil 1/4 cup
- Granulated swerve sweetener 3 tbsp.
- Dark chocolate chips, sugar-free (like lily's) 1 cup
- Egg yolks 4 large
- Coconut flakes 1 cup

- Kosher salt 1/2 tsp.
- Walnuts roughly chopped 3/4 cup.

Directions

1. Heat oven up to 350° and line a parchment paper on a baking sheet. In a large mixing bowl, whisk together butter, coconut oil, sweetener, egg yolks and salt; stir in walnuts, coconut, and chocolate chips.

2. Drop spoonfuls of batter onto the prepared baking sheet. Place in the oven and bake for 15 mins until golden,

12. No-Bake Coconut Crack Bars
Prep. Time: 2 minutes

Cook Time: 3 minutes

Servings: 20

The serving size is 1 square

Nutrition as per serving:

108kcal / 11g fat / 2g carbs / 2g fiber /2g protein = 0g net carbs

Ingredients

- Coconut flakes unsweetened & Shredded 3 cups
- Coconut oil, melted 1 cup
- Maple syrup, monk fruit sweetened 1/4 cup (or any liquid sweetener of preference)

Directions

1. Line parchment paper on an 8 x 10-inch pan or an 8 x 8-inch pan and put aside. Or use a loaf pan.

2. Combine unsweetened shredded coconut, melted coconut oil, maple syrup (monk fruit sweetened) in a big mixing bowl and mix till you get a thick batter. If you find it crumbling, add a tsp. of water or a bit of extra syrup.

3. Transfer the coconut mixture to the lined pan. Press firmly with slightly wet hands into place. Chill until firmed. Cut into bars & enjoy!

13. Candied Pecans

Prep. Time: 5 minutes

Cook Time: 1 minute

Servings: 16 Servings

The serving size is 1 Serving

Nutrition as per serving:

139kcal / 15g fat / 3g carbs / 2g fiber / 2g protein = 1g net carbs

Ingredients

• Granulated sweetener divided 1 1/2 cups

• Vanilla extract 1 tsp

• Water 1/4 cup

• Cinnamon 1 tbsp.

• Raw pecans 3 cups

Directions

1. Over medium flame, heat a skillet or large pan.

KETO DIET COOKBOOK FOR BEGINNERS BY CASEY BLACK

2. Add 1 cup of the granulated sweetener, vanilla extract and water, and stir until fully mixed. Let it heat up, stirring in between.

3. Once the sweetener is fully melted, include your pecans. Stir around the pecans ensuring every nut is equally coated in the liquid mixture. Keep occasionally stirring till the sweetener starts to set on the pecans. Take off from the heat. Leave for 2 to 3 minutes.

4. Brea apart the pecans with a wooden spoon before they set together.

5. When cooled, mix with the granulated sweetener that was reserved earlier and cinnamon. Store in a sealed container.

14. Sugar-Free Flourless Cookies

Prep. Time: 2 minutes

Cook Time: 10 minutes

Servings: 14 cookies

The serving size is 1 Cookie

Nutrition as per serving:

101kcal / 9g fat / 3g carbs / 1g fiber / 5g protein = 3g net carbs

Ingredients

For the original style:

• Almond butter 1 cup

• Egg 1 large

• Granulated sweetener, stevia blend monk fruit, 3 /4 cup

For the egg-free style:

- Almond butter smooth 1 cup

- Chia seeds, ground 3-4 tbsp.

- Granulated sweetener, stevia blend monk fruit 3/4 cup

Directions

1. Heat the oven up to 350 degrees. Place parchment paper on a cookie sheet or a baking tray.

2. In a big mixing bowl, add all the ingredients and blend until well combined. When using the egg-free recipe, begin with 3 tbsps. of grounded chia seeds. Add an extra tbsp. if the mixture is still too thin.

3. Using your hands or a cookie scoop, shape small balls and place them 3 to 4 inches apart on the baking tray. Make into cookie shape by pressing down with a fork. Bake until cookies are beginning to get a golden brown color but still soft, or for 8 to 10 minutes. Take out from the oven, allowing to cool until firm but soft and chewy.

15. Salted Caramel Fudge

Prep. Time: 5 minutes

Cook Time: 5 minutes

Servings: 24 servings

The serving size is 1 fudge cup

Nutrition as per serving:

148kcal / 15g fat / 4g carbs / 2g fiber / 4g protein = 2g net carbs

Ingredients

- Cashew butter 2 cups
- Keto maple syrup 1/4 cup
- Coconut oil 1/2 cup

Directions

1. Line muffin liners in a mini muffin tin of 24-count and put aside.
2. Combine all the ingredients on a stovetop or in a microwave-safe dish and heat till melted.
3. Take off from heat and beat very well till a glossy, smooth texture remains.
4. Split the fudge mixture equally in the lined muffin tin. Chill for about 30 minutes, till firm.

16. Healthy Kit Kat Bars

Prep. Time: 5 minutes

Cook Time: 5 minutes

Servings: 20 Bars

The serving size is 1 Bar

Nutrition as per serving:

149kcal / 12g fat / 4g carbs / 2g fiber / 7g protein = 2g net carbs

Ingredients

- Keto granola 2 cups
- Almond butter (or any seed or nut butter) 1 cup
- Mixed seeds 1/2 cup
- Coconut oil 1/4 cup
- Mixed nuts 1/2 cup
- Dark chocolate chips, 1 1/2 cups
- Sticky sweetener 1/2 cup

Directions

1. Mix the mixed nuts, keto granola, and seeds in a big bowl. Put aside.
2. Melt the keto chocolate chips on the stovetop or in a microwave-safe dish. Include almond butter, coconut oil, and sticky sweetener. Heat until well combined.
3. Add the melted chocolate mixture onto the dry and combine until fully unified.
4. Shift the kit kat mixture to a pan of 10 x 10-inch lined with parchment. With a spatula, smooth out to a uniform layer. Chill for about 30 minutes, then slice into bars.

Notes: keep refrigerated

17. Healthy No-Bake Keto Cookie Bars

Prep. Time: 5 minutes

Cook Time: 25 minutes

Servings: 12 servings

The serving size is 1 Bar

Nutrition as per serving:

149kcal / 5g fat / 10g carbs / 6g fiber / 10g protein = 4g net carbs

Ingredients

For the cookie

- Almond flour blanched 1 1/2 cups

- Coconut flour 1/4 cup

- Cinnamon, a pinch

- Protein powder, vanilla flavor (optional) 2 scoops

- Granulated sweetener (like

- Sticky sweetener, keto-friendly, 1/2 cup

- Monk fruit sweetener) 2 tbsp.

- Vanilla extract 1/2 tsp

- Cashew butter (or any nut butter) 1/2 cup

- Sticky sweetener, keto-friendly, 1/2 cup

- Almond milk 1 tbsp.

For the protein icing

- Protein powder,

- Vanilla flavor 3 scoops

- Granulated sweetener, keto-friendly 1-2 tbsp. + for sprinkling 1/2 tsp

- Almond milk, (for batter) 1 tbsp.

For the coconut butter icing

- Coconut butter melted 4-6 tbsp.

- Sticky sweetener, 2 tbsp.

- Almond milk 1 tbsp.

Directions

1. Preparing sugar cookie base

2. Place tin foil in a baking pan of 8 x 8 inches and put aside.

3. Mix the protein powder, flours, granulated sweetener and cinnamon in a big mixing bowl, and put aside.

4. Melt the sticky sweetener with cashew butter on a stovetop or a microwave-proof bowl. Stir in the vanilla extract and add to the dry mixture. Beat superbly until fully combined. If the batter formed is too thick, add a tablespoon of almond milk with a tablespoon and mix well until desired consistency.

5. Pour the batter into the lined baking sheet and press tightly in place. Scatter the ½ teaspoon of keto-friendly granulated sweetener and chill for about 15 minutes until they are firm. Then add an icing of choice and chill for 30 minutes more to settle the icing before slicing.

6. Preparing the icing(s)

7. Mix all ingredients of the icings (separately) and, using almond milk, thin down the mixture till a very thick icing is formed.

18. Keto Chocolate Bark with Almonds and Bacon

Prep. Time: 30 minutes

Servings: 8 servings

The serving size is 1/8 of the recipe

Nutrition as per serving:

157kcal /12.8g fat / 4g protein / 7.5g fiber / 12.7g carbs = 5.2g net carbs

Ingredients

- Sugar-free Chocolate Chips 1 bag (9 oz.)
- Chopped Almonds 1/2 cup
- Bacon cooked & crumbled2 slices

Directions

1. In a microwave-safe bowl, melt the chocolate chips on high in 30 seconds intervals, stirring every time until all chocolate is melted.
2. Include the chopped almonds into the melted chocolate and mix.
3. Line a baking sheet with parchment and pour the chocolate mixture on it in a thin layer of about 1/2 inch.
4. Immediately top the chocolate with the crumbled bacon and press in with a flat spoon.
5. Chill for around 20 minutes or till the chocolate has solidified. Peel the parchment away from the hardened chocolate and crack it into eight pieces. Keep refrigerated.

Chapter 2- Chaffles

1. Basic chaffle recipe

Prep. Time: 5 minutes

Cook Time: 5 minutes

Servings: 1 chaffle

The serving size is 1 chaffle

Nutrition as per serving:

291kcal / 23g fat / 1g carbs / 0g fiber / 20g protein = 1g net carbs

Ingredients

- Sharp cheddar cheese shredded 1/2 cup

- Eggs 1

Directions

1. Whisk the egg.

2. In the waffle maker, assemble 1/4 cup of shredded cheese.

3. Top the cheese with beaten egg.

4. Top with the remainder 1/4 cup of cheese.

5. Cook till it's golden and crispy. It will get crispier as it cools.

2. Keto Oreo Chaffles

Prep. Time: 15 minutes

Cook Time: 8 minutes

Servings: 2 full-size chaffles or 4 mini chaffles

The serving size is 2 chaffles

Nutrition as per serving:

381kcal / 14.6g fat / 14g carbs / 5g fiber / 17g protein = 9g net carbs

Ingredients

• Sugar-Free Chocolate Chips 1/2 cup

• Butter 1/2 cup

• Eggs 3

• Truvia 1/4 cup

• Vanilla extract 1tsp.

• For Cream Cheese Frosting

• Butter, room temperature 4 oz.

• Cream Cheese, room temperature 4 oz.

• Powdered Swerve 1/2 cup

• Heavy Whipping Cream 1/4 cup

• Vanilla extract 1tsp.

Directions

1. Melt the butter and chocolate for around 1 minute in a microwave-proof dish. Stir well. You really ought to use the warmth within the chocolate and butter to melt most of the clumps. You have overheated the chocolate; when you microwave, and all is melted, it means you have overheated the chocolate. So grab yourself a spoon and begin stirring. If required, add 10 seconds, but stir just before you plan to do so.

2. Put the eggs, vanilla and sweetener, in a bowl and whisk until fluffy and light.

3. In a steady stream, add the melted chocolate into the egg mix and whisk again until well-combined.

4. In a Waffle Maker, pour around 1/4 of the mixture and cook for 7 to-8 minutes until it's crispy.

5. Prepare the frosting as they are cooking.

6. Put all the frosting ingredients into a food processor bowl and mix until fluffy and smooth. To achieve the right consistency, include a little extra cream.

7. To create your Oreo Chaffle, spread or pipe the frosting evenly in between the two chaffles.

8. The waffle machine, do not overfill it! It will create a giant mess and ruin the batter and the maker, utilizing no more than 1/4 cup of the batter.

9. Leave the waffles to cool down a bit before frosting. It is going to help them to remain crisp.

10. To make the frosting, use room-temp butter and cream cheese.

3. Glazed Donut Chaffle

Prep. Time: 10 mins

Cook Time: 5 mins

Servings: 3 chaffles

The serving size is 1 chaffle

Nutrition as per serving:

312kcal / 15g fat / 6g carbs / 1g fiber / 9g protein = 5g net carbs

Ingredients

For the chaffles

- Mozzarella cheese shredded ½ cup
- Whey protein isolates Unflavored 2 tbsp.
- Cream Cheese 1 oz.
- Swerve confectioners (Sugar substitute) 2 tbsp.
- Vanilla extract ½tsp.
- Egg 1
- Baking powder ½tsp.

For the glaze topping:

- Heavy whipping cream2 tbsp.
- Swerve confectioners (sugar substitute) 3-4 tbsp.
- Vanilla extract ½tsp.

Directions

1. Turn on the waffle maker.

2. In a microwave-proof bowl, combine the cream cheese and mozzarella cheese. Microwave at 30-second breaks until it is all melted and stir to combine completely.

3. Include the whey protein, baking powder, 2 tbsp. Keto sweetener to the melted cheese, and work with your hands to knead until well combined.

4. Put the dough in a mixing bowl, and whisk in the vanilla and egg into it to form a smooth batter.

5. Put 1/3 of the mixture into the waffle machine, and let it cook for 3 to 5 minutes.

6. Repeat the above step 5 to make a total of three chaffles.

7. Whisk the glaze topping ingredients together and drizzle on top of the chaffles generously before serving.

4. Keto Pumpkin Chaffles

Prep. Time: 2 mins

Cook Time: 5 mins

Servings: 2 chaffles

The serving size is 2 chaffles

Nutrition as per serving: (without toppings)

250kcal / 15g fat / 5g carbs / 1g fiber / 23g protein = 4g net carbs

Ingredients

- Mozzarella cheese, shredded ½ cup

- Egg, beaten 1 whole

- Pumpkin purée 1 ½ tbsp.

- Swerve confectioners ½tsp.

- Vanilla extract ½tsp.

- Pumpkin pie spice ¼tsp.

- Pure maple extract ⅛tsp.

- For topping- optional

- roasted pecans, cinnamon, whip cream and sugar-free maple syrup

Directions

1. Switch on the Waffle Maker and begin preparing the mixture.

2. Add all the given ingredients to a bowl, except for the mozzarella cheese, and whisk. Include the cheese and combine until well mixed.

3. Grease the waffle plates and put half the mixture into the middle of the plate. Cover the lid for 4- to 6 minutes, based on how crispy Chaffles you like.

4. Take it out and cook the second one. Serve with all or some mix of toppings, like sugar-free maple syrup, butter, roasted pecans, and a dollop of whipping cream or ground cinnamon dust.

5. Cream Cheese Chaffle with Lemon Curd

Prep. Time: 5 minutes

Cook Time: 4 minutes

Additional Time: 40 minute

Servings: 2-3 serving

The serving size is 1 chaffle

Nutrition as per serving:

302 kcals / 24g fat / 6g carbs / 1g fiber / 15g protein = 5g net carbs

Ingredients

- One batch keto lemon curd (recipe here)
- Eggs 3 large
- Cream cheese softened 4 oz.
- Lakanto monkfruit (or any low carb sweetener) 1 tbsp.

- Vanilla extract 1tsp.

- Mozzarella cheese shredded 3/4 cup

- Coconut flour 3 tbsp.

- Baking powder 1tsp.

- Salt 1/3tsp.

- Homemade keto whipped cream (optional) (recipe here)

Directions

1. Prepare lemon curd according to Directions and let cool in the refrigerator.

2. Turn on the waffle maker and grease it with oil.

3. Take a small bowl, put coconut flour, salt and baking powder. Combine and put aside.

4. Take a large bowl, put cream cheese, eggs, vanilla and sweetener. With an electric beater, beat until foamy. You may see chunks of cream cheese, and that is okay.

5. Include mozzarella cheese into the egg mixture and keep beating.

6. Pour the dry ingredients into the egg mixture and keep mixing until well blended.

7. Put batter into the preheated waffle machine and cook.

8. Take off from waffle machine; spread cooled lemon curd, top with keto whipped cream and enjoy.

6. Strawberries & Cream Keto Chaffles

Prep. Time: 25 minutes

Cook Time: 10 minutes

Servings: 8 chaffles

The serving size is 1 chaffle

Nutrition as per serving:

328cals / 12g fat / 8g carbs / 4g fiber / 6g protein = 4g net carbs

Ingredients

- Cream cheese 3 oz.

- Mozzarella cheese, shredded 2 cups

- Eggs, beaten 2

- Almond flour 1/2 cup

- Swerve confectioner sweetener 3 tbsp. + 1 tbsp.

- Baking powder 2tsps

- Strawberries 8

- Whipped cream 1 cup (canister - 2 tbsp. Per waffle)

Directions

1. In a microwavable dish, add the mozzarella and cream cheese, cook for 1 minute, mixing well. If the cheese is all melted, then go to the next step. Else cook for another 30 seconds stirring well.

2. Take another bowl, whisk eggs, including the almond flour, 3 tbsp. of keto sweetener, and baking powder.

3. Include the melted cheese mixture into the egg and almond flour mixture and combine well. Carefully add in 2 strawberries coarsely chopped. Chill for 20 minutes.

4. Meanwhile, slice the unused strawberries and mix with 1 tbsp. of Swerve. Chill.

5. Take out the batter from the refrigerator after 20 minutes. Heat the waffle iron and grease it.

6. Put 1/4 cup of the batter in the mid of the heated waffle iron. Ensuring the waffles are small makes it easier to remove from the waffle maker.

7. Transfer to a plate when cooked and cool before adding whipped cream and topping with strawberries.

This recipe gave me eight small waffles.

7. Keto Peanut Butter Cup Chaffle

Prep. Time: 2 minutes

Cook Time: 5 minutes

Servings: 2 Chaffles

The serving size is 1 chaffle + filling

Nutrition as per serving:

264kcal / 21.6g fat / 7.2g carbs / 2g fiber / 9.45g protein = 4.2g net carbs

Ingredients

For the Chaffle

- Heavy Cream 1 tbsp.
- Vanilla Extract 1/2 tsp
- Egg 1
- Cake Batter Flavor 1/2 tsp
- Unsweetened Cocoa 1 tbsp.
- Coconut Flour 1 tsp
- Lakanto Powdered Sweetener 1 tbsp.
- Baking Powder 1/4 tsp

For Peanut Butter Filling

- Heavy Cream 2 tbsp.
- All-natural Peanut Butter 3 tbsp.
- Lakanto Powdered Sweetener 2 tsp

Directions

1. Preheat a waffle maker.
2. Combine all the chaffle ingredients in a small mixing bowl.
3. Put half of the chaffle batter into the middle of the waffle machine and cook for 3 to 5 minutes.
4. Cautiously remove and duplicate for the second chaffle. Leave chaffles for a couple of minutes to let them crisp up.
5. Prepare the peanut butter filling by blending all the ingredients together and layer between chaffles.

8. Vanilla Chocolate Chip

Prep. Time: 1 minute

Cook Time: 4 minutes

Servings: 1 serving

The serving size is 1 large or 2 mini chaffle

Nutrition as per serving:

297.6 kcal. / 20.1g fat / 5.2g carbs / 1.5g fiber / 22.2g protein = 3.9g net carbs

Ingredients

- Mozzarella shredded 1/2 cup

- Eggs 1 medium

- Granulated sweetener keto 1 tbsp.

- Vanilla extract 1 tsp

- Almond meal or flour 2 tbsp.

- Chocolate chips, sugar-free 1 tbsp.

Directions

1. Mix all the ingredients in a large bowl.

2. Turn on the waffle maker. When it is heated, grease with olive oil and put half the mixture into the waffle machine. Cook for 2 to 4 minutes, then take out and repeat. It will make 2 small-chaffles per recipe.

3. Enjoy with your favorite toppings.

9. Chaffle Churro

Prep. Time: 10 minutes

Cook Time: 6-10 minutes

Servings: 2

The serving size is 4 churros

Nutrition as per serving:

189 kcals / 14.3g fat / 5.g carbs / 1g fiber / 10g protein = 4g net carbs

Ingredients

- Egg 1

- Almond flour 1 Tbsp.

- Vanilla extract ½ tsp.

- Cinnamon divided 1 tsp.

- Baking powder ¼ tsp.
- Shredded mozzarella ½ cup.
- Swerve confectioners (or any sugar substitute) 1 Tbsp.
- Swerve brown sugar (keto-friendly sugar substitute) 1 Tbsp.
- Butter melted 1 Tbsp.

Directions

1. Heat the waffle iron.

2. Combine the almond flour, egg, vanilla extract, baking powder, ½ tsp of cinnamon, swerve confectioners' sugar and shredded mozzarella in a bowl, and stir to combine well.

3. Spread half of the batter equally onto the waffle iron, and let it cook for 3 to 5 minutes. Cooking for more time will give a crispier chaffle.

4. Take out the cooked chaffle and pour the remaining batter onto it. Close the lid and cook for about 3 to 5 minutes.

5. Make both the chaffles into strips.

6. Put the cut strips in a bowl and drizzle on melted butter generously.

7. In another bowl, stir together the keto brown sugar and the leftover ½ tsp of cinnamon until well-combined.

8. Toss the churro chaffle strips in the sugar-cinnamon mixture in the bowl to coat them evenly.

10. Keto Cauliflower Chaffles Recipe

Prep. Time: 5 minutes

Cook Time: 4 minutes

Servings: 2 chaffles

The serving size is 2 chaffles

Nutrition as per serving:

246kcal / 16g fat / 7g carbs / 2g fiber / 20g protein = 5g net carbs

Ingredients

- Riced cauliflower 1 cup
- Garlic powder 1/4tsp.
- Ground black pepper 1/4tsp.
- Italian seasoning 1/2tsp.
- Kosher salt 1/4tsp.
- Mozzarella cheese shredded 1/2 cup
- Eggs 1
- Parmesan cheese shredded 1/2 cup

Directions

1. In a blender, add all the ingredients and blend well. Turn the waffle maker on.
2. Put 1/8 cup of parmesan cheese onto the waffle machine. Ensure to cover up the bottom of the waffle machine entirely.
3. Cover the cheese with the cauliflower batter, then sprinkle another layer of parmesan cheese on the cauliflower mixture. Cover and cook.
4. Cook for 4 to 5 minutes, or till crispy.
5. Will make 2 regular-size chaffles or 4 mini chaffles.
6. It freezes well. Prepare a big lot and freeze for the future.

11. Zucchini Chaffles

Prep. Time: 10 minutes

Cook Time: 5 minutes

Servings: 2 chaffles

The serving size is 1 chaffle

Nutrition as per serving:

194kcal / 13g fat / 4g carbs / 1g fiber / 16g protein = 3g net carbs

Ingredients

- Zucchini, grated 1 cup

- Eggs, beaten 1

- Parmesan cheese shredded 1/2 cup

- Mozzarella cheese shredded 1/4 cup
- Dried basil, 1tsp. Or fresh basil, chopped 1/4 cup
- Kosher Salt, divided 3/4tsp.
- Ground Black Pepper 1/2tsp.

Directions

1. Put the shredded zucchini in a bowl and Sprinkle salt, about 1/4tsp on it and leave it aside to gather other ingredients. Moments before using put the zucchini in a paper towel, wrap and press to wring out all the extra water.

2. Take a bowl and whisk in the egg. Include the mozzarella, grated zucchini, basil, and pepper 1/2tsp of salt.

3. Cover the waffle maker base with a layer of 1 to 2 tbsp. of the shredded parmesan.

4. Then spread 1/4 of the zucchini batter. Spread another layer of 1 to 2 tbsp. of shredded parmesan and shut the lid.

5. Let it cook for 4 to 8 minutes. It depends on the dimensions of your waffle machine. Normally, once the chaffle is not emitting vapors of steam, it is nearly done. For the greatest results, let it cook until good and browned.

6. Take out and duplicate for the next waffle.

Will make 4 small chaffles or 2 full-size chaffles in a Mini waffle maker.

12. Keto Pizza Chaffle

Prep. Time: 10 minutes

Cook Time: 30 minutes

Servings: 2 servings

The serving size is 1 chaffle

Nutrition as per serving:

76 kcal / 4.3g fat / 4.1g carbs / 1.2g fiber / 5.5g protein = 3.2g net carbs

Ingredients

- Egg 1
- Mozzarella cheese shredded 1/2 cup
- Italian seasoning a pinch
- Pizza sauce No sugar added 1 tbsp.
- Toppings – pepperoni, shredded cheese (or any other toppings)

Directions

- Heat the waffle maker.
- Whisk the egg, and Italian seasonings in a small mixing bowl, together.
- Stir in the cheese, leaving a few tsps. for layering.
- Layer a tsp of grated cheese onto the preheated waffle machine and allow it to cook for about 30 seconds.
- It will make a crispier crust.
- Pour half the pizza mixture into the waffle maker and allow to cook for around 4 minutes till it's slightly crispy and golden brown!

- Take out the waffle and make the second chaffle with the remaining mixture.

- Spread the pizza sauce, pepperoni and shredded cheese. Place in Microwave and heat on high for around 20 seconds and done! On the spot Chaffle PIZZA!

13. Crispy Taco Chaffle Shells

Prep. Time: 5 minutes

Cook Time: 8 minutes

Servings: 2 chaffles

The serving size is 1 chaffle

Nutrition as per serving:

258kcal / 19g fat / 4g carbs / 2g fiber / 18g protein = 2g net carbs

Ingredients

- Egg white 1

- Monterey jack cheese shredded 1/4 cup

- Sharp cheddar cheese shredded 1/4 cup

- Water 3/4 tsp

- Coconut flour 1 tsp

- Baking powder 1/4 tsp

- Chili powder 1/8 tsp

- Salt a pinch

Directions

1. Turn on the Waffle iron and lightly grease it with oil when it is hot.

2. In a mixing bowl, mix all of the above ingredients and blend to combine.

3. Pour half of the mixture onto the waffle iron and shut the lid. Cook for 4 minutes without lifting the lid. The chaffle will not set in less than 4 minutes.

4. Take out the cooked taco chaffle and put it aside. Do the same process with the remaining chaffle batter.

5. Put a muffin pan upside down and assemble the taco chaffle upon the cups to make into a taco shell. Put aside for a few minutes.

6. When it is firm, fill it with your favorite Taco Meat fillings. Serve.

Enjoy this delicious keto crispy taco chaffle shell with your favorite toppings.

Chapter 3- Keto Cakes and Cupcakes

1. Chocolate Cake with Chocolate Icing

Prep. Time: 10 minutes

Cook Time: 25 minutes

Servings: 9 slices

The serving size is 1 slice

Nutrition as per serving:

358kcal / 33g fat / 11g carbs / 6g fiber / 8g protein = 5g net carbs

Ingredients

- Coconut flour 3/4 cup
- Granular sweetener 3/4 cup
- Cocoa powder 1/2 cup
- Baking powder 2tsps
- Eggs 6
- Heavy whipping cream 2/3 cup
- Melted butter 1/2 cup
- For chocolate icing
- Heavy whipping cream 1 cup
- Keto granular sweetener 1/4 cup
- Vanilla extracts 1tsp.
- Cocoa powder sifted 1/3 cup

Directions

1. Heat the oven up to 350F.
2. Oil a cake pan of 8x8.
3. In a large mixing bowl, put all the cake ingredients to blend well with an electric mixer or a stand mixer.
4. Transfer the batter to the oiled pan and put in the heated oven for 25 minutes or till a toothpick inserted in the center comes out clean.
5. Take out from the oven. Leave to cool fully before icing.
6. Prepare the Icing

7. With an electric mixer, beat the whipping cream until stiff peaks form. Include the cocoa powder, swerve, and vanilla. Keep beating until just combined.

8. Spread the icing evenly all over the cake and serve. Keep any remains in the refrigerator.

2. 4 Ingredients Cheesecake Fluff

Prep. Time: 10 minutes

Servings: 6

The serving size is ½ cup

Nutrition as per serving:

258kcal / 27g fat / 4g carbs / 0g fiber / 4g protein = 4g net carbs

Ingredients

- Heavy Whipping Cream1 Cup
- Cream Cheese, Softened 1 Brick (8 oz.)
- Lemon Zest 1 tsp.
- Keto-friendly Granular Sweetener 1/2 Cup

Directions

1. Prepare the Fluff

2. Put the heavy cream in a bowl of a stand mixer and beat until stiff peaks begin to form. An electric beater or a hand beater can also be used.

3. Transfer the whipped cream into a separate bowl and put aside

4. To the same stand mixer bowl, add the cream cheese (softened), sweetener, zest, and whisk until smooth.

5. Now add the whipped cream to the cream cheese into the mixer bowl. Fold with a spatula gently till it is halfway combined. Finish whipping with the stand mixer until smooth.

6. Top with your fave toppings and serve.

3. Mug Cake Peanut Butter, Chocolate or Vanilla

Prep. Time: 4 minutes

Cook Time: 1 minute

Servings: 1

The serving size is 1 mug cake

Nutrition as per serving:

(For mug cake with almond flour: chocolate flavor and no chocolate chips)

312 kcal / 7 carbs/ 28g fat / 12g protein/4g fiber = 3 net carbs

(Peanut butter flavor and no chocolate chips)

395 kcal / 8 carbs /35g fat / 15g protein/4g fiber = 5 net carb

(Vanilla flavor and no chocolate chips)

303 kcal / 5 carbs/ 28g fat / 11g protein /2g fiber = 3 net carb

Ingredients

- Butter melted 1 Tbsp.

- Almond flour 3 Tbsp. or Coconut flour 1 Tbsp.

- Granular Sweetener 2 Tbsp.

- Sugar-free Peanut butter 1 Tbsp. (For Peanut Butter flavor)

- Cocoa powder 1 Tbsp. (For Chocolate flavor)

- Baking powder ½ tsp.

- Egg, beaten 1

- Sugar-free Chocolate Chips 1 Tbsp.

- Vanilla few drops

Directions

For Vanilla flavor

1. In a microwave-proof coffee mug, heat the butter for 10 seconds to melt in the microwave.

2. Include the almond flour or coconut flour, baking powder, sweetener, beaten egg and vanilla. Combine well.

3. For 60 seconds, microwave on high, ensuring not to overcook; otherwise, it will come out dry. Sprinkle keto chocolate chips on top if preferred or stir in before cooking.

For Chocolate flavor

In a microwave-proof coffee mug, heat the butter for 10 seconds to melt in the microwave. Include the almond flour or coconut flour, cocoa powder, sweetener, baking powder, beaten egg and vanilla. Combine well. For 60 seconds, microwave on high, ensuring not to overcook; it will come out dry. Sprinkle keto chocolate chips on top if preferred.

For Peanut Butter flavor

1. In a microwave-proof coffee mug, heat the butter for 10 seconds to melt in the microwave.
2. Include the almond flour or coconut flour, baking powder, sweetener, beaten egg and vanilla. Combine well. Stir in peanut butter. For 60 seconds, microwave on high, ensuring not to overcook; otherwise, it will come out dry. Sprinkle keto chocolate chips on top if preferred.

Directions for Baking: Bake in an oven-safe small bowl. Bake in the oven for 15 to 20 minutes at 350.

4. Chocolate Coconut Flour Cupcakes

Prep. Time: 10 minutes

Cook Time: 25 minutes

Servings: 12 cupcakes

The serving size is 1 cupcake

Nutrition as per serving:

268 kcal / 22g fat / 6g carbs / 3g fiber / 6g protein = 3g net carbs

Ingredients

For Cupcakes:

- Butter melted 1/2 cup
- Cocoa powder 7 tbsp.
- Instant coffee granules 1 tsp (optional)
- Eggs at room temperature 7
- Vanilla extracts 1 tsp
- Coconut flour 2/3 cup
- Baking powder 2 tsp
- Swerve sweetener 2/3 cup
- Salt 1/2 tsp
- Hemp milk or unsweetened almond milk 1/2 cup (+more)

For Espresso Buttercream:

- Hot water 2 tbsp.
- Instant coffee or instant espresso powder 2 tsp
- Whipping cream 1/2 cup

- Butter softened 6 tbsp.
- Cream cheese softened 4 oz.
- Swerve powdered sweetener 1/2 cup

Directions

For Cupcakes:

1. Heat the oven up to 350F and line silicone liners or parchment on a muffin tin.
2. Mix together the cocoa powder, melted butter, and espresso powder in a large mixing bowl,
3. Include the vanilla and eggs and whisk until well combined. Now add in the coconut flour, baking powder, salt and sweetener, and mix until smooth.
4. Pour the almond milk in and stir. If the batter is very thick, add in 1 tbsp. of almond milk at a time to thin it out. It should not be pourable but of scoopable consistency.
5. Scoop the batter equally among the prepared muffin tins and put in the oven's center rack, baking for 20-25 minutes. Check the cupcakes with a tester inserted into the center comes out clean, then cupcakes are done. Leave to cool in the pan for 5 to 10 minutes, and then cool completely on a wire rack.

For Buttercream:

1. Dissolve the coffee in hot water. Put aside.
2. Whip cream using an electric mixer until stiff peaks are formed. Put aside.
3. Beat cream cheese, butter, and sweetener all together in a medium mixing bowl until creamy. Include coffee mixture and mix until combined. fold in the whipped cream Using a rubber spatula carefully till well combined.
4. Layer frosting on the cooled cupcakes with an offset spatula or a knife.

5. Low-carb red velvet cupcakes/ cake

Prep. Time: 15-30 minutes

Cook Time: 20-25 minutes

Servings: 12 slice

The serving size is 1 slice

Nutrition as per serving:

193kcals / 12g fat / 6.4g carbs / 1g fiber / 5.9g protein = 5.4g net carbs

Ingredients

- Almond flour 1+ 3/4 cups
- Swerve confectioner sweetener (not substitutes) 2/3 cup
- Cocoa powder 2 tbsp.
- Baking powder 2tsp.
- Baking soda 1/2tsp.
- Eggs 2
- Full fat coconut milk 1/2 cup + 2 tbsp.
- Olive oil 3 tbsp.
- Apple cider vinegar 1 tbsp.
- Vanilla extract 1 tbsp.
- Red food coloring 2 tbsp.

For frosting

- Cream cheese at room temperature 1 container (8 oz.)
- Butter softened 2 ½ tbsp.
- Swerve confectioner sweetener 1 cup

- Coconut milk 2 ½ tbsp.

- Vanilla extract 1tsp.

- Salt 1/8tsp.

**Double Frosting for Layer Cake

Directions

1. Preheat oven to 350 degrees

2. In a large mixing bowl, add the wet ingredients, eggs, milk, vanilla extract, olive oil, apple cider vinegar and food coloring. Blend until smooth.

3. Now sift together the cocoa powder, Swerve Confectioner, baking powder and baking soda, add to the wet ingredients, and incorporate it into the batter with an electric mixer or a hand whisk.

4. Lastly, sift in the almond flour. Moving the flour back and forth with a whisk will speed up the process significantly. Fold the sifted flour gently into the batter till smooth and all is well incorporated. Use the batter immediately.

5. To make Cupcakes: Scoop batter into the muffin liners, fill only up to 2/3 of liner -do not over-fill. Ensure the oven is heated, put in the oven for 15 minutes at 350 degrees, and then turn the muffin tin in 180 degrees and cook for an extra 10 minutes. (Bear in mind, oven times vary occasionally - humidity and altitude can impact things, so watch closely as they may need a few minutes more or even less).

6. Take out from the oven, do not remove from pan and set aside to cool completely.

7. For Layer Cake: 2 Layer- line parchment paper in two cake pans (8 inches each) and oil the sides. Transfer batter to both pans evenly. Use a wet spatula to spread

the batter smoothly. Apply the same process for three layers, but using thinner pans as dividing the batter three ways-every layers will become thin.

8. Place pans into oven for 20-25 minutes baking at 350 degrees. Cautiously turn the pans 180 degrees halfway through baking and cover lightly with a foil. At 20 to 25 minutes, take out the pans; they will be a bit soft. Set them aside to cool completely. When they are cool, take a knife and run it around the side of the pan and turn them over carefully onto a plate or cooling rack and leave them for an extra 5 to 10 minutes before icing.

9. Meanwhile, prepare. Blend the softened butter and cream cheese together With an electric beater. Include milk and vanilla extract and beat again. Lastly, sift in the Swerve, salt mixing well one last time. If you want a thicker frosting, chill it in the refrigerator. Or adding more Swerve will give a thicker texture or add more milk to make it thinner. * For a layer cake, double the frosting recipe.

10. Spread or pipe frosting onto cupcakes, sprinkle some decoration if desired and enjoy!! To frost layer cake, it is simpler to first chill the layers in the freezer. Then frost and pile each layer to end frost the sides and top.

Keep any leftovers in a sealed box and refrigerate. Enjoy!

6. Vanilla Cupcakes

Prep. Time: 5 minutes

Cook Time: 20 minutes

Servings: 10 Cupcakes

The serving size is 1 cupcake

Nutrition as per serving:

153kcal / 13g fat / 4g carbs / 2g fiber / 5g protein = 2g net carbs

Ingredients

- Butter 1/2 cup
- Keto granulated sweetener 2/3 cup
- Vanilla extract 2 tsp
- Eggs whisked * See notes 6 large

- Milk of choice ** See notes 2 tbsp.

- Coconut flour 1/2 cup

- Baking powder 1 tsp

- Keto vanilla frosting 1 batch

Directions

1. Heat the oven up to 350F/180C. Place muffin liners in a 12-cup muffin tin and oil 10 of them.

2. Beat the butter, salt, sugar, eggs and vanilla extract together in a big mixing bowl when combined-well include the milk and mix until blended.

3. In another bowl, sift the baking powder and coconut flour together. Add the wet ingredients to the dry and mix until combined.

4. Pour the batter equally into the ten muffin cups, filling up to ¾ full. Place the cupcakes on the middle rack and bake for 17 to 20 minutes until the muffin top springs back to touch

5. Remove the muffin pan from the oven, set it aside to cool for 10 minutes, and then cool completely on a wire rack. Frost, when cooled.

7. Healthy Flourless Fudge Brownies

Prep. Time: 5 minutes

Cook Time: 20 minutes

Servings: 12 servings

The serving size is 1 Brownie

Nutrition as per serving:

86kcal / 5g fat / 5g carbs / 3g fiber / 7g protein = 2g net carbs

Ingredients

- Pumpkin puree 2 cups

- Almond butter 1 cup

- Cocoa powder 1/2 cup

- Granulated sweetener (or liquid stevia drops) 1/4 cup

For the Chocolate Coconut Frosting

- Chocolate chips 2 cups

- Coconut milk canned 1 cup

- For the chocolate protein frosting

- Protein powder, chocolate flavor 2 scoops

- Granulated sweetener 1-2 tbsp.

- Seed or nut butter of choice 1-2 tbsp.

- Milk or liquid *1 tbsp.

For the Cheese Cream Frosting

- Cream cheese 125 grams

- Cocoa powder 1-2 tbsp.

- Granulated sweetener of choice 1-2 tbsp.

Directions

1. For the fudge brownies

2. Heat the oven up to 350 degrees, oil a loaf pan or small cake pan and put aside.

3. Melt the nut butter in a small microwave-proof bowl. In a big mixing bowl, put in the pumpkin puree, dark cocoa powder, nut butter, and combine very well.

4. Transfer the mixture to the oiled pan and put in preheated oven for around 20 to 25 minutes or until fully baked. Remove from the oven, set aside to cool completely. When cooled, apply the frosting and chill for about 30 minutes to settle.

Preparing the cream cheese or protein frosting:

1. In a big mixing bowl, mix together all the ingredients and beat well. With a tablespoon. keep adding dairy-free milk till a frosting consistency is reached.

2. For the coconut chocolate ganache

3. In a microwave-proof bowl, combine all the ingredients and heat gradually until just mixed- whisk till a glossy and thick frosting remains.

8. Healthy Keto Chocolate Raspberry Mug Cake
Prep. Time: 1 minute

Cook Time: 1 minute

Servings: 1 serving

The serving size is 1 mug cake

Nutrition as per serving:

152kcal / 8g fat / 13g carbs / 8g fiber / 7g protein = 5g net carbs

Ingredients

- Coconut flour 1 tbsp.

- Granulated sweetener of choice 1 tbsp.

- Cocoa powder 2 tbsp.

- Baking powder 1/4 tsp

- Sunflower seed butter (or any seed or nut butter) 1 tbsp.

- Pumpkin puree 3 tbsp.

- Frozen or fresh raspberries 1/4 cup

- Coconut milk unsweetened 1-2 tbsp.

Directions

1. In a microwave-proof mug, put in the dry ingredients and stir well.

2. Add in the rest of the ingredients, except for milk and raspberries, and combine until a thick batter is formed.

3. Stir in the raspberries and add one tbsp. of milk. Add extra milk if the batter gets too thick. Place in microwave and cook for 1 to 2 minutes. Should come out gooey in the center. If you overcook, it will become dry.

Oven Directions

1. Heat oven up to 180C.

2. Oil an oven-proof ramekin. Add the prepared batter and put in the oven for 10-12 minutes, or until done.

9. Keto Avocado Brownies

Prep. Time: 10 minutes

Cook Time: 30 minutes

Servings: 12 squares

Nutrition as per serving:

155kcal / 14g fat / 13g carbs / 10g fiber / 4g protein = 2.8g net carbs

Ingredients

- Avocado, mashed 1 cup

- Vanilla 1/2 tsp

- Cocoa powder 4 tbsp.

- Refined coconut oil (or ghee, butter, lard, shortening) 3 tbsp.

- Eggs 2

- Lily's chocolate chips melted 1/2 cup (100 g)

Dry Ingredients

- Blanched almond flour 3/4 cup

- Baking soda 1/4 tsp

- Baking powder 1 tsp

- Salt 1/4 tsp

- Erythritol 1/4 cup (see sweetener note *1)

- Stevia powder 1 tsp (see sweetener note *1)

Directions

1. Heat the oven up to 350F/ 180C.

2. Sift together the dry ingredients in a small bowl and stir.

3. Place the Peeled avocados in a food processor and process until smooth.

4. One by one, add all the wet ingredients into the food processor, processing every few seconds

5. Now include the dry ingredients into the food processor and blend until combined.

6. Line a parchment paper in a baking dish (of 12"x8") and transfer the batter into it. Spread evenly and put in the heated oven. Cook for 30 minutes or the center springs back to touch. It should be soft to touch.

7. Remove from oven, set aside to cool fully before cutting into 12 slices.

10. Low Carb-1 minute Cinnamon Roll Mug Cake

Prep. Time: 1 minute

Cook Time: 1 minute

Servings: 1 serving

The serving size is 1mug

Nutrition as per serving:

132kcal / 4g fat / 6g carbs / 2g fiber / 25g protein = 4g net carbs

Ingredients

- Protein powder, vanilla flavor 1 scoop
- Baking powder 1/2 tsp
- Coconut flour 1 tbsp.
- Cinnamon 1/2 tsp
- Granulated sweetener 1 tbsp.
- Egg 1 large

- Almond milk, unsweetened 1/4 cup

- Vanilla extract 1/4 tsp

- Granulated sweetener 1 tsp

- Cinnamon 1/2 tsp

For the glaze

- Coconut butter melted 1 tbsp.

- Almond milk 1/2 tsp

- Cinnamon a pinch

Directions

1. Oil a microwave-proof mug. In a small bowl, add the protein powder, coconut flour, baking powder, sweetener, cinnamon and mix well.

2. Add in the egg and stir into the flour mixture. Include the vanilla extract and milk. If the batter is too dry, keep adding milk until a thick consistency is reached.

3. Pour this batter into the oiled mug. Sprinkle extra cinnamon and keto granulated sweetener over the top and swirl. Place in microwave and cook for 60 seconds, or till the center is just cooked. Do not overcook, or it will come out dry. Drizzle the glaze on top and enjoy!

4. Prepare glaze by mixing all ingredients and use.

11. Double Chocolate Muffins

Prep. Time: 10 minutes

Cook Time: 15 minutes

Servings: 12 muffins

The serving size is 1 muffin

Nutrition as per serving:

280 kcal / 27g fat / 7g carbs / 4g fiber / 7g protein = 3g net carbs

Ingredients

- Almond flour 2 cup
- Cocoa powder unsweetened 3/4 cup
- Swerve sweetener 1/4 cup
- Baking powder 1 1/2 tsp.
- Kosher salt 1 tsp.
- Butter melted 1 cup (2 sticks)
- Eggs 3 large
- Pure vanilla extract 1 tsp.
- Dark chocolate chips, sugar-free (like lily's) 1 cup

Directions

1. Heat oven up to 350° and line cupcake liners in a muffin tin. In a big bowl, stir together almond flour, Swerve, cocoa powder, salt and baking powder. Include eggs, melted butter and vanilla and mix until combined.
2. Stir in the chocolate chips.

3. Pour batter equally in muffin cups and bake for 12 minutes or until the muffin top springs back to touch.

Chapter 4- Keto Fat Bombs

1. Cheesecake Fat Bombs

Prep. Time: 5 minutes

Servings: 24Fat Bombs

The serving size is 1 Fat Bomb

Nutrition as per serving:

108kcal / 12g fat / 1g carbs / 1g fiber / 1g protein = 0g net carbs

Ingredients

- Heavy Cream 4 oz.

- Cream cheese at room temperature 8 oz.

- Erythritol 2-3 tbsp.

- Coconut oil or butter 4 oz.

- Vanilla extracts 2tsp.

KETO DIET COOKBOOK FOR BEGINNERS BY CASEY BLACK

- Baking chocolate or coconut for decorating

Directions

1. In a big mixing bowl, add all the ingredients and mix for 1-2 minutes with an electric mixer until well combined and creamy.

2. Spoon mixture into an unlined or lined mini cupcake tin. Chill for 1-2 hours in the refrigerator or freezer for about 30 minutes.

3. Take out from the cupcake tins and store them in a sealed container. It can be refrigerated for up to two weeks.

2. Brownie Fat Bombs

Prep. Time: 15 minutes

Servings: 16 fat bombs

The serving size is 2 fat bombs

Nutrition as per serving:

174 kcal / 16g fat / 4g carbs / 2g fiber / 3g protein = 2g net carbs

Ingredients

- Ghee 1/4 cup

- Cocoa butter 1 oz.

- Vanilla extract 1/2 tsp

- Salt 1/4 tsp

- Raw cacao powder 6 tbsp.

- Swerve Sweetener powdered 1/3 cup

- Water 2 tbsp.

- Almond butter 1/3 cup
- Nuts, chopped (optional) 1/4 cup

Directions

1. melt the cocoa butter and ghee together In a heat-safe bowl placed over a pot of simmering water,
2. Add in the sweetener, cacao powder, salt and vanilla extract. This mixture will be smooth and thin.
3. Stir in the water and beat the mixture till it thickens to the consistency of a thick frosting.
4. Mix in the nut butter with a rubber spatula. The mixture will look like cookie dough. Mix in the coarsely chopped nuts.
5. Shape into 1 inch sized balls (will make about 16) and chill until firm.

3. Coffee Fat Bombs

Prep. Time: 10 minutes

Servings: 8 Fat Bombs

The serving size is 1 Fat Bomb

Nutrition as per serving:

140 kcal / 14g fat / 4g carbs / 2g fiber / 1.5g protein = 2g net carbs

Ingredients

- Cream Cheese, Full-fat 8 Oz.
- Butter Unsalted, ½ cup (1 Stick)
- Instant Coffee 1 to 2 Tbsps.
- Chocolate Chips, Low Carb, heaped ¼ Cup

- Confectioners Erythritol heaped ⅓ Cup
- Cocoa Powder, Unsweetened 1½ Tbsp.

Directions

1. In a large bowl, place the butter and cream cheese (both should be at room temperature)
2. Combine them with an electric mixer until smooth.
3. Then include all the remaining ingredients in the bowl, blending until well-combined
4. Scoop out the batter with a tablespoon or a cookie scoop to make around 12 bombs. Place them on a baking sheet lined with parchment. Chill for about 3 hours.

4. Peanut Butter Fat Bombs

Prep. Time: 10 minutes

Servings: 12 fat bombs

The serving size is 1/2 fat bomb

Nutrition as per serving:

247 kcal / 24.3g fat / 3.2g carbs / 1.2g fiber / 3.6g protein = 2g net carbs

Ingredients

For fat bomb

- Natural peanut butter (no sugar) 3/4 cup
- Coconut oil (melted) 1/2 cup
- Vanilla extract 1 tsp.
- Liquid stevia 3 – 4 drops

- Sea salt 1/4 tsp.

For Ganache

- Coconut oil 6 tbsp.

- Cocoa powder 1 tbsp.

- Liquid stevia 1 – 2 drops

Directions

1. Mix the peanut butter, coconut oil, vanilla extract, salt, and liquid stevia together in a small mixing bowl, beat until creamy and smooth.

2. Line muffin paper cups in a six-cup-muffin tray. Fill each cup with about 3 tbsp. of the peanut butter mixture.

3. Refrigerate for about 1 hour to solidify.

4. Meanwhile, beat together the ingredients for Ganache until it's silky.

5. Drizzle about one tbsp. of the chocolate ganache on every fat bomb.

6. Chill for about 30 minutes and enjoy.

5. Cream Cheese Pumpkin Spiced Fat Bombs

Prep. Time: 10 minutes

Servings: 12 Fat Bombs

The serving size is 1 Fat Bomb

Nutrition as per serving:

80 kcal / 7.5g fat / 2g carbs / 0.25g fiber / 1.5g protein = 1.75g net carbs

Ingredients

- Pure pumpkin ⅔ cup

- Pumpkin pie spice ½ tsp
- Cream cheese, full-fat 8 oz.
- Butter melted 3 tbsps.
- Confectioner's erythritol 3 tbsps.

Directions

1. Place all the ingredients in a large bowl and mix with an electric mixer until combined.
2. Make 12 equal-sized balls from the dough. Place paper liners in a mini-muffin tin and place the PB cookie dough in the muffin tin.
3. Chill for a minimum of 2 hours

Note:

If the pumpkin pie spice is not available, make some with the following ingredients

¼ tsp cinnamon, a pinch of (each) - nutmeg, cloves, ginger and allspice.

6. Brownie Truffles

Prep. Time: 5 minutes

Cook Time: 5 minutes

Servings: 20 Truffles

The serving size is 1 Truffle

Nutrition as per serving:

97kcal / 8g fat / 5g carbs / 3g fiber / 4g protein = 2g net carbs

Ingredients

- Sticky sweetener, keto-friendly 1/2 cup of choice

- Homemade Nutella 2 cups
- Coconut flour 3/4 cup (or almond flour 1 ½ cup)
- Chocolate chips, sugar-free 2 cups

Directions

1. Combine the coconut/almond flour, sticky sweetener and chocolate spread in a big mixing bowl. Add a bit more syrup or liquid; if the mixture is too thick, it should become a creamy dough.

2. Place parchment paper on a large plate. Shape into small balls with your hands, and set on the plate. Chill.

3. Melt the sugar-free chocolate chips. Take the truffles from the refrigerator. Immediately, coat each truffle with the melted chocolate, making sure all are evenly coated.

4. Set back on the lined

5. Plate and chill until firm.

7. Coconut Strawberry Fat Bombs

Prep. Time: 10 minutes

Servings: 20 fat bombs

The serving size is 1fat Bomb

Nutrition as per serving:

132kcals / 14.3g fat / 0.9g carbs / 0g fiber / 0.4g protein = 0.9g net carbs

Ingredients

For Coconut base:

- Coconut cream 1 1/2 cups
- Coconut oil (melted) 1/2 cup
- Stevia liquid 1/2 tsp.
- Lime juice 1 tbsp.

For Strawberry topping:

- Fresh chopped strawberries 2 oz.
- Coconut oil (melted) 1/2 cup
- Liquid stevia 5 – 8 drops

Directions

Prepare the coconut base:

1. In a high-speed blender, place all the coconut base ingredients and blend them completely until combined and smooth.
2. Distribute the mixture evenly into an ice cube tray, muffin tray, or a candy mold, leaving room for the topping.
3. Chill in the freezer to set for about 20 minutes.

For the Strawberry topping:

1. In a blender, put all the ingredients for the strawberry topping, then blend until smooth.
2. When the base is set, spoon the strawberry mixture equally over each one.
3. Refrigerate the fat bombs for about 2 hours and enjoy.

8. Raspberry & White Chocolate Fat Bombs
Prep. Time: 5 minutes

Servings: 10-12 fat bombs

The serving size is 1 fat Bomb

Nutrition as per serving:

153kcal / 16g fat / 1.5g carbs / 0.4g fiber / 0.2g protein = 1.2g net carbs

Ingredients

- Cacao butter 2 oz.
- Coconut oil 1/2 cup
- Raspberries freeze-dried 1/2 cup
- Erythritol sweetener, powdered (like swerve) 1/4 cup

Directions

1. Place paper liners in a 12-cup muffin pan.

2. In a small pot, heat the cacao butter and coconut oil on low flame until melted completely. Take off the pot from heat.

3. Blend the freeze-dried raspberries in a blender or food processor, or coffee grinder.

4. Include the sweetener and powdered berries into the pot, stirring to dissolve the sweetener.

5. Distribute the mixture evenly between the muffin cups. Don't worry if the raspberry powder sinks to the bottom. Just stir the mixture when pouring them into each mold to distribute the raspberry powder in each mold.

6. Chill until hard. Enjoy.

9. Almond Joy Fat Bombs (3 Ingredients)

Prep. Time: 2 minutes

Cook Time: 3 minutes

Servings: 24 cups

The serving size is 1 cup

Nutrition as per serving:

72kcal / 8g fat / 6g carbs / 4g fiber / 2g protein = 2g net carbs

Ingredients

- Coconut butter softened 1/4 cup
- Chocolate chips, sugar-free, divided 20 oz.
- Almonds 24 whole

Directions

1. Place muffin liners in a 24-cup mini muffin tin and put them aside.

2. Melt 3/4 of the sugar-free chocolate chips in a microwave-proof bowl. Distribute the chocolate mixture equally into all the muffin liners. Also, scrape down all the chocolate coated on the sides. Chill until firm.

3. When the chocolate is hard, spoon in the melted coconut butter evenly into every chocolate cup, leaving room for chocolate filling on top. Add in more softened coconut butter if needed.

4. Melt the rest of the chocolate chips and with it, cover each of the chocolate coconut cups. Place an almond on top of each cup and chill until firm.

10. Pecan pie fat bombs

Prep. Time: 15 minutes

Servings: 18 balls

The serving size is 2 balls

Nutrition as per serving

121 kcal / 12g fat / 3.8g carbs / 2.9g fiber / 2g protein = 0.9g net carbs

Ingredients

- Pecans, (or any nut) 1½ cup s
- Coconut butter, ¼ cup
- Coconut shredded ½ cup
- Chia seeds 2 tbsp.
- Pecan butter (or any nut butter) 2 tbsp.
- Flax meal 2 tbsp.
- Coconut oil 1tsp.
- Hemp seeds 2 tbsp.
- Vanilla extract ½tsp.
- Cinnamon 1½tsp.
- Kosher salt ¼tsp.

Directions

1. Add the ingredients altogether in a food processor. Process for a minute or two to break down the mixture. First, it will become powdery. Then it will stick together but remain crumbly.

2. Continue to process until the oils begin to expel a bit, and the mixture will begin to stick together easily –be cautious not to process excessively, or you will have nut butter.

3. Using a tablespoon or small cookie scooper, scoop to make equal pieces of the mixture. Roll them into balls with your hands placing them all on a large plate. Chill for about 30 mins.

4. Keep in a sealed container or a zip-lock bag in the freezer or refrigerator.

11. PB. Cookie Dough Fat Bomb

Prep. Time: 10 minutes

Servings: 12 Fat Bombs

The serving size is 1 Fat Bomb

Nutrition as per serving:

135kcal / 11g fat / 5g carbs / 3.5g fiber / 4g protein = 1.5g net carbs

Ingredients

- Lily's chocolate chips ⅓ cup
- Almond flour, superfine 1 cup
- Natural peanut butter 6 tbsps.
- Confectioner's erythritol 2 tbsps.
- Coconut oil (melted) 1 tbsps.
- Vanilla extract 1 tsp
- Salt, a pinch

Directions

1. Place all the ingredients in a large bowl and mix with a spoon until crumbly.

2. Form a dough ball with your hands.

3. Line parchment paper on a baking sheet. Scoop out equal-sized 12 cookie dough fat bombs.

4. Chill for about an hour

5. Once they are done setting, keep in a sealed bag in the fridge.

Conclusion

When going on a ketogenic diet, one retains modest protein consumption but increases their fat intake. The transition to a low-carb diet brings your body into a ketosis state, where fat is used for energy compared to carbohydrates.

It takes some time for fats to decompose through the digestive tract and delay the decomposition of the carbohydrates into sugar, maintain our blood sugar concentrations steady and allow us to feel satiated longer. Based on observational evidence, incorporating a tablespoonful of coconut oil into your diet every day may also result in lower weight.

You may also need to monitor the portion sizes, but as fat is intrinsically pleasing, having one for breakfast will help deter eating during meals.

When consuming high-fat meals, including keto fat bombs, you will further encourage weight reduction by decreasing appetite for the next meal. Be it fat bombs or cheesy waffles or any other hi fat low-carb dessert, they are a dieter's dream come true.

Following the keto diet can positively impact one's brain function.

Advantages of the ketogenic diet and fat bombs.

Keto fat bombs may be seen as a way to reduce sugar habits.

Ketogenic fat bombs are simple to produce, easy to keep, and easy to eat; they often need fewer ingredients than other foods.

Ketogenic fat bombs are tasty and have a broad variety of low-carb recipes.

Ketogenic fat bombs are quick to produce, are easy to store, and are ready to consume at any time.

In this book, you will find the best and easy to prepare keto cakes, chaffles, and yummy high-fat recipes that will fulfill your cravings for desserts after meals or snacks when you don't feel too hungry. Enjoy these recipes by yourself, or even better, share the joy with family and friends!

Intermittent Fasting for Women Over 60

The Science-Based Program for Seniors to Conquer and Keep a Young Body, Reset Your Metabolism and Activate Autophagy Above 60's

[11 Anti-Aging Exercises Included]

By

Casey Black

Table of Contents

INTRODUCTION

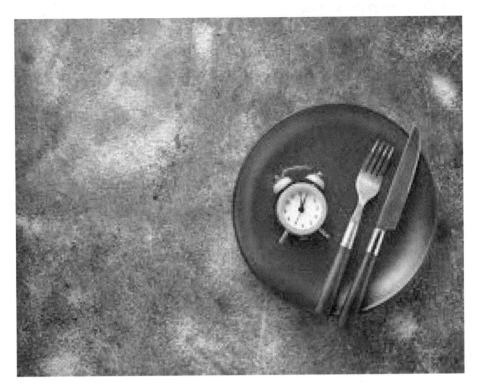

What exactly does intermittent fasting refer to? Almost all of us are familiar with the word fasting. The reasons people fast vary from one group to another. For some, it is a religious practice; they sacrifice food to commit to prayer. Others have no reason; they just lack food. In past societies, people would go out to the fields to work, and eat only when they rested.

Intermittent fasting is not among the fasting practices described above. It is neither a religious practice, nor is it driven by the lack of time or food - it is a choice. It is best described as an eating pattern that alternates between eating periods and fasting periods, with each period lasting a predetermined amount of time. For example, the 16:8 method has a fasting period of 16 hours and an eating period of 8 hours.

Note that it is not a diet but an eating pattern. Less is said about the foods you should eat, but more emphasis is put on when you eat them. Does this mean you can eat whatever you want? Unfortunately not. Just like anything else in life, you're going to get out what you put in. Clean eating is one of the three factors in the tripod to fat burning success. Does this mean you must live on chicken and broccoli? No of course not. We are humans and I believe in enjoying life, but as you already know moderation is the key here.

It is important to know that IF isn't some program that popped up from somewhere, will trend for a while, and disappear like most weight loss programs do. It has been around for a long time and has been popular for many years (even if you are learning about it just now). It is one of the leading health and fitness trends in the world today.

PART ONE

Knowledge (The Science-Based Program for Seniors to Conquer and Keep a Young Body)

How Fat is Stored & Burnt

Intermittent fasting has been tried and found to be a powerful fat burning and weight loss tool. But how exactly does it work? Before delving into how IF works it's important to understand some key factors:

➢ How the body stores energy

➢ How the body uses energy

➢ Your hormones role in this process

The body is either in a state of storing energy or burning energy. There is no middle ground.

What does this mean? Well basically if you're not burning glucose (sugar) you're storing it as either glycogen or fat. Does this mean you need to be constantly working out? Short answer- no. In fact, exercise is only 10% - 15% of the weight loss equation (more about that later). Your body burns energy in a variety of different ways. Even when you're stationary doing absolutely nothing your body expends energy as it completes functions required for living. This is what RMR or BMR refers to. However, even though your cells might be using glucose and burning energy, any excess will be stored. This would count as a state of storage.

Wait! If we're either storing sugar or burning it, logic would dictate less food and more exercise equals weight loss. It seems straight forward, right? If you're reading this you have most likely tried this approach to no avail. You either saw results in the beginning only to have them come to a grinding halt or you put it all back on when you returned to your normal lifestyle.

So, how do I lose weight then?? To get a better picture we need to understand two principles:

1.   How glucose (sugar) is stored and burned, or used for energy.

2.   Our hormone's role in this process

How is energy stored?

The body can store energy in two ways; glycogen and fat.

Food (yum) is broken down into a variety of different macronutrients through digestion. These macronutrients are absorbed into the bloodstream and transported throughout the body to our cells to use for various functions. For example, Carbohydrates are broken down into Glucose (sugar), absorbed by the blood stream and sent to cells to use for energy. However, if there is excess glucose in the bloodstream (high blood sugar), it will be stored as glycogen through a process called Glycogenesis. The body can only store so much glycogen. Once these stores are full any excess glucose is stored as fat through a process called Lipogenesis.

How is energy used?

When our cells require more energy than the bloodstream can provide (low blood sugar) glycogen is turned back into glucose through a process called glycogenolysis. Our glycogen stores are slowly emptied to raise our blood sugar levels back to normal. When these stores are empty, fat will be broken down for energy in a process called lipolysis. Now we're burning fat Wahoo!

Summary

➤ Excess glucose will be turned into glycogen for storage, triggered by high blood sugar

➤ Once glycogen stores are full, excess glucose will be turned into fat for storage

➤ When blood sugar levels drop, glycogen will be turned back into glucose and added to the bloodstream

➤ When glycogen stores are emptied, fat will be broken down and released into the bloodstream for energy

Now you have a rough idea of how and why the body stores and uses energy, we will look at some key hormones that control this process.

Why Low-Calorie Diets Don't Work

Have you ever tried lowering your calories to lose weight? Did it work long term? Could you keep the weight you lost off? If you're reading this book, my guess is that it didn't, and you're not alone. Data from the UK show 1 in 124 obese women get results using this method, meaning the nutrition guidelines some professionals are following have a 99.5% fail rate. A quick goggle of what happened to the contestants on the hit TV series "The Biggest Loser" should be enough to put you off this method. This show is a classic example of why moving more and eating less only works in the short term, if at all. There is a reason there are few reunion shows. So why are low calorie diets flawed?

A study on 14 contestants on the biggest loser show revealed some alarming results six years after filming had finished. The initial results were impressive but as the study showed, they were short lived. Below are results of some of the factors tested.

Weight

- Average weight before filming: 328 lb./ 148 kg

- Average weight after 30 weeks on the show: 199 lb./ 90 kg

- Average weight six years after final: 290 lb./131 kg

As you can see, contestants lost a massive amount of weight during filming, but struggled to maintain the weight loss over a long period of time.

One of the 14 who participated in the study managed to keep the weight off. That's over a 95% fail rate! So why is this?

Check out the results below showing contestants Resting metabolic rate (RMR).

Resting Metabolic Rate

RMR reflects the amount of energy or calories the body burns to stay alive without movement.

In some places this is measured in BMR or basal metabolic rate.

RMR is responsible for around 70% of your entire metabolism which is why the results below are shocking.

- Average RMR before filming: 2,607 kcal burned / day.

- Average RMR after 30 weeks on the show: 1,996 kcal burned / day.

- Average RMR six years after final weigh-in: 1,903 kcal burned / day.

As you can see, even though contestants put around 70% of their initial weight back on, their RMR did not raise back to its levels pre- filming. It stayed around 700 calories lower a day! This means to lose the same amount of weight second time round; contestants would need to eat 700 less calories than they did on the show. Considering the original diet consists of 1200 - 1500 calories with 90 minutes of exercise six days a week. This would be near impossible.

So why did the contestants RMR stay so low even when they put the weight back on?

Metabolic adaptation

I mentioned BMR (basal metabolic rate) and RMR (resting metabolic rate) earlier. These both refer to how much energy (calories) your body uses to live without action and make up roughly 70% of your entire metabolism. When you sit in caloric deficit, the bodies BMR/RMR will slowly drop as it enters starvation mode, meaning it will burn less calories. Basically, your metabolism slows down. This is an important reaction through times of famine. The body doesn't want to use its stored energy, and naturally uses incoming energy sparingly. This is not beneficial when the aim is everlasting, sustainable weight loss. When you start dieting in this manner and increase your exercise you will generally only see results at the start before your body's metabolism adjusts for the lack of food. Once it adjusts, your results become stagnant and often times after frustration people give up and all the weight comes piling back on. If you're lucky your RMR/BMR will rise with the weight gain, ensuring you only end up putting back on what you lost, but constant yo-yo dieting could lead to a lower metabolism meaning you will struggle to lose weight and could even end up the heaviest you've ever been!

So, if eating too little causes this, you're probably wondering how not eating at all over a period of time could be any better right? Keep reading to see why.

Intermittent fasting vs Low calorie diets

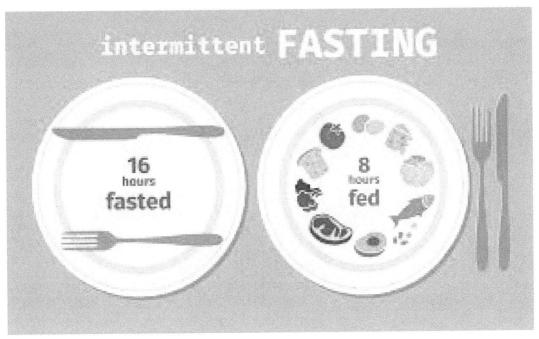

Low calorie diets simply don't cause the hormone adaptations fasting does. Remember those hormones we covered earlier in the book? They are the key to weight loss and your salvation. Remember how we need the help of hormones such as glucagon and HGH to stimulate the liver and fat cells to break down stored energy? As we now know they're triggered by low blood sugar levels. This is accomplished during the fasted period. Other hormones I haven't mentioned for simplicity's sake are also stimulated during this window to prevent metabolism drops associated with low calorie diets. Low calorie diets still include eating, and every time we eat our blood sugar levels are going to rise which triggers.........Insulin! As you now know, insulin is a storage hormone. So even though you might be consuming low calories, your lowered metabolism plus this little guy equals stored fat. Nothing turns off HGH like high blood sugar levels and insulin which ruins your chance to maintain muscle mass.

Summary

- Low calorie dieting could ruin your metabolism making maintainable weight loss near impossible

- Maintainable weight loss relies heavily on hormone adaptation

- Fasting stimulates key hormones for metabolism retention, muscle preservation, and fat burning

WHAT YOU SHOULD WEIGH

Before you embark on a fasting program for weight loss, let me help you establish what you should weigh. For many people, women in particular, the figure we think of as "ideal" is far removed from what is realistic, or even healthy. I could go on and blame the media or the fashion industry. We all know that argument and, yes, it's partly true.

Ironically, where I learned about fasting in India, the thought of using fasting to get slim would be abhorrent, as being skinny is associated with poverty and lower social castes. Fasting should never be used to strive for a body that's slimmer than is healthy – the size zero craze being a case in point. The less body fat you have to lose, the more you need to ensure that fasting is not over- done since weight loss is a guaranteed side-effect.

BODY MASS INDEX (BMI)

Healthy weight ranges are especially useful if you're already light for your frame

– you've probably heard of BMI, which gives an indication of how healthy your current weight is in proportion to your height. The formula for calculating BMI is:

$$BMI = weight (kg) \div height (m)2$$

(in other words, your weight in kilograms divided by your height in meters squared).

If math isn't your strong point, you can find out your BMI using an online calculator.

A healthy BMI is between 18.5 and 24.9. Although many celebrities have a BMI below 18.5, this simply isn't healthy. Some studies suggest that the ideal BMI is 23 for men and 21 for women – particularly if it's a long and healthy life you're after.

However, if your BMI is, say, 25 you won't become magically healthier by losing 450g (1lb) and dieting down to a BMI of 24.9. In fact, it's perfectly possible for someone with a BMI of 27 to be much healthier than someone with a BMI of 23. That's because BMI doesn't take your body fat, waist circumference, eating habits or lifestyle into account. An example of this could be a professional rugby player who's heavier than average simply because he or she is very muscular. There's nothing unhealthy about having lots of muscle, but the BMI scale might say he or she is overweight or even obese. In contrast, a chain-smoker who lives on diet drinks and never exercises can have a so-called "healthy" BMI. Who do you think is healthier?

A BMI of 30 or above is considered "obese". A 2008 study by researchers at the Mayo Clinic in the USA, involving over 13,000 people, found that 20.8 percent of men and 30.7 percent of women were obese according to the BMI scale. But when they used the World Health Organization gold standard definition of obesity – measuring body fat percentage – 50 percent of the men and 62.1 percent of the women were classified as obese. (In other words, you can have a healthy BMI and an unhealthy level of body fat.) What this means is that the athlete who's unfairly classed as "obese" is the exception rather than the rule. Unless you're an avid weight-lifter or sportsperson, or you have an extremely physical job, the BMI scale isn't likely to tell you that you need to lose weight if you don't. If your BMI is well over 25, don't worry. Medical experts agree that losing 5–10 percent of your starting weight is a sensible and realistic initial goal that will have lasting health benefits.

Therefore, when it comes to the BMI scale, it is worth calculating your BMI before deciding on a weight loss goal, especially if you only have a little weight to lose, but it definitely shouldn't be the only thing you think about.

BODY FAT PERCENTAGE

What's great about monitoring your body fat percentage is that it gives you a better understanding of what's going on inside your body as you lose weight. Sustainable weight loss is best achieved through a combination of good nutrition and an active lifestyle. The thing is, when you start exercising more, you often gain muscle mass.

It can be demotivating to step onto the scales and see that your overall weight hasn't changed in spite of all your hard work. But because muscle is denser than fat, you can look slimmer and achieve health benefits without actually losing weight. To track changes in your body fat, you need to invest in body composition scales which enable you to track your progress by measuring changes in your muscle mass, body fat and hydration. Gyms often have high- quality versions of these scales if you don't want to buy your own.

Body composition scales are also helpful because if you notice that your muscle mass is decreasing as rapidly as your body fat, this suggests that you've cut your energy intake too dramatically. For most people, it's realistic to lose 450–900g (1–2lb) of body fat per week. If you're losing much more than this, the chances are you're eating into your muscle mass. Body composition scales can alert you to this before you've risked damaging your health.

In women, it's normal for hydration levels to fluctuate along with the menstrual cycle. Again, measuring weight alone doesn't enable you to track these changes. By using the body composition scales at a similar time of day, and recording changes throughout the month, you can get a clearer understanding of the times you're gaining body fat, and when it's simply a matter of fluid retention.

Sophisticated body composition monitors also enable you to track abdominal fat. Remember, not all fat is created equal, and abdominal fat is concentrated around your vital organs, posing the biggest health risk. You can be a "healthy" weight, and have high levels of abdominal fat – being aware of this can give you the motivation you need to address your eating habits and activity level.

The scales use a weak electric current to differentiate between fat, muscle, fluid and bone – we won't go into too much detail here as different brands have different features. As a guide, if you're an ordinary adult, and not an athlete or aspiring fitness model, you should be aiming for the following body fat percentages:

AGE	MALE	FEMALE
20–39	8–20%	21–33%
40–59	11–22%	23–34%
60+	13–25%	24–36%

WHY TRADITIONAL DIETING MAKES YOU HUNGRY

Going on a traditional diet without adequate energy intake for long periods of time can make your metabolic rate plummet and your appetite soar. Say you reduce your calories to below 1,000 a day for a number of weeks to fit into a party dress, the chances are you'll feel hungry and fed up much of the time, and as soon as the party starts, you'll dive head first into all the foods you've been avoiding, re-gaining that lost weight in no time! This, in a nutshell, sums up the seesaw of the diet industry.

The real trick is to keep your body feeling fuller for longer. I'm not talking about choosing one ready-meal over another, it's about understanding how to manage hunger so you naturally eat less most of the time. Please note, I don't say all of the time. Special events and over-indulging every now and then are good for the soul.

In tandem with a good diet overall, fasting can be used to retrain your hunger without the need for appetite suppressants or dodgy supplements. When you begin to fast, you will feel hungry at your usual meal times. However, if you choose not to eat at that time, the peaks and troughs of hunger start to level out. All this happens without a decrease in metabolic rate. It doesn't take a genius to recognize that if you feel hungry less often, you'll eat less and therefore lose weight. There's a biological explanation for this. Feelings of hunger and satiety (feeling full) are controlled by two main hormones produced within the body, ghrelin (even the word sounds hungry) and leptin. This dynamic duo of hormones has a powerful effect on how much food you eat and how much of what you've consumed you "burn off".

GHRELIN

This hormone seems pretty straightforward. When your stomach's empty, it sends out some ghrelin to tell an area of your brain, the hypothalamus, that you ought to be eating. You then feel ravenous. But research published in the American Journal of Physiology suggests that ghrelin levels also rise in anticipation of eating – you get hungry partly because you're expecting a meal, not just because you have an empty stomach.

On a traditional diet, you get a peak of ghrelin before every meal – but because you don't eat as much as you'd really like to, you never feel fully satisfied. When you're fasting, your ghrelin levels still rise, but anecdotal evidence suggests that over time your body finds this sensation easier to get used to, probably because of the changes in your meal patterns. There's also a theory that a nutritionally poor diet (think additive-packed "diet" meals) sends ghrelin rocketing faster than a nutrient-dense plan like the ones I recommend.

LEPTIN

This hormone is a little more complicated. You'll sometimes hear leptin referred to as a "master regulator" of fat metabolism. There are even whole diet books devoted to it.

Leptin is made by the fat cells – put simply, the more fat you have, the more leptin is produced. Like ghrelin, it sends a signal to the hypothalamus, but with the opposite effect. Leptin is supposed to maintain your body fat at a healthy level by telling you to stop eating when you start to gain too much fat. We all know it doesn't really work like that in practice – if it did, no one would be overweight. So, what happens?

Well, leptin also increases when you overeat – especially stodgy, carbohydrate-rich meals. This is because its release is triggered by insulin, which responds to an increase in blood glucose after a meal. So, if you're constantly eating without a proper break, your leptin levels will always be high. At first this is good – it should signal to your brain that it's time to put down that muffin – but it can lead to a very dangerous vicious circle. The theory is that, over time, too much leptin leads to the brain becoming resistant to its effects. As your brain stops recognizing what leptin is trying to tell it, you end up feeling hungry all the time, and are never satisfied by even the biggest meal.

WHY MOST DIETS FAIL

This probably isn't the first book about weight loss you've ever read. I often say I've been down the diet road myself so many times that I could be a tour guide. If you're asking yourself why fasting is going to be any different, here are the facts you need to know:

• "Yo-yo" dieting is the bane of many people's lives, but even if you've lost and gained weight countless times, recent research has shown that it's possible to lose weight safely without messing up your metabolism.

• Burning off more calories than you eat is the only way to lose weight – and the simple truth is that you will lose weight if you manage to keep the number of calories you eat below the amount you burn off… boring but true.

There are hundreds of different ways to create a calorie deficit – as evidenced by the huge diet book, diet shake, diet bar and "miracle" weight-loss supplement industry. But there are two main reasons why diets never tend to live up to their expectations, especially as you get closer to your goal weight:

1   *Traditional diet misrepresent the calories in/calories out equation*.

We've all heard that 450g (1lb) of fat is roughly equal to 3,500 calories, so the traditional calorie-counting approach is to cut calories by 500–1,000 per day in order to lose 450–900g (1–2lb) per week. The trouble is, as you get slimmer you become lighter and that actually reduces the number of calories you burn at rest (your basal metabolic rate). So, in traditional weight-loss plans, weight loss is initially rapid but tends to slow down over time, even if you maintain that original calorie deficit. This can be very demotivating.

2   *It's sticking to your chosen approach that's often the hard part.*

Even if you get your calories exactly right, how boring does counting every calorie get? Demotivation – either as a result of not seeing the numbers on the scales going down as quickly as they were, or boredom – can lead to lapses, which slow down the rate of weight loss even further. When you go back to your old eating habits – surprise, surprise – you'll gain all the weight back, and a little more, as a result of the natural dip in basal metabolic rate (calorie burn) caused by your initial weight loss.

PART TWO

Action (Reset Your Metabolism)

HOW FASTING MAKES A DIFFERENCE

FASTING MAY BOOST METABOLIC RATE

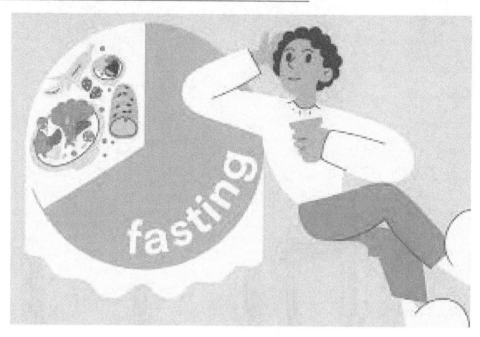

You're probably thinking, "If I start starving myself, won't that be worse for my metabolism?" First of all, fasting is not starving yourself, and don't worry that eating less often will damage your metabolism. Losing weight naturally slows your basal metabolic rate (the number of calories you burn at rest) in proportion to the amount of weight you lose, no matter which method you use. This is because your daily energy (calorie) needs are directly related to your age, height, gender and weight, in particular your lean body mass (muscle). It doesn't mean that eating more often will fire up your metabolism.

You'll hear over and over again that after a night of sleep, your metabolism has ground to a halt and you need to eat breakfast to stoke your metabolic fire. The idea that "breakfast boosts metabolism" is simply not true – it hasn't been backed up by research at all. The breakfast myth is based on the "thermic effect of food". Around 10 percent of our calorie burn comes from the energy that we use to digest, absorb and assimilate the nutrients in our meals. Roughly speaking, if you eat a 350-calorie breakfast, you'll burn 35 calories in the process. But notice that you've eaten 315 extra calories to burn that 35. No matter what time of day you eat, you'll burn off around 10 percent of the calories in your food through the thermic effect of food. So, whether you eat your breakfast at 7am, 10am or never, if you eat roughly the same amount and types of food overall, its effect on your metabolism will be the same.

In fact, all the research on fasting seems to show that eating less often could actually boost your metabolic rate. In one British study conducted at the University of Nottingham, a two-day fast boosted participants' resting metabolic rate by 3.6 percent. In another study by the same research group, 29 healthy men and women fasted for three days. After 12–36 hours, there was a significant increase in basal metabolic rate, which returned to normal after 72 hours. The exact mechanisms for why this happens aren't clear.

FASTING INCREASES FAT BURN

What is clear is that more of the calories you use for fuel during fasting come from your fat stores. Scientists can estimate what proportion of your energy is coming from fats and carbohydrates by measuring the amount of oxygen inhaled and the amount of carbon dioxide exhaled in your breath. The higher the proportion of oxygen to carbon dioxide, the more fat you're burning. As part of the same Nottingham study, findings proved that the proportion of energy obtained from fat rose progressively over 12–72 hours, until almost all the energy being used was coming from stored fat. This is incredible news really!

We're so often told to "breakfast like a king, lunch like a prince and dine like a pauper" with a view to becoming healthy, wealthy and wise. This is usually explained by telling us that breakfast kick-starts the metabolism – but it turns out that eating breakfast doesn't boost your fat-burning potential at all. In a small study on breakfast-eaters – published in the British Journal of Nutrition – a 700-calorie breakfast inhibited the use of fat for fuel throughout the day. Put simply, when we eat carbohydrates, we use it for fuel, and this prevents our bodies tapping into our stubborn stored fat. Constant grazing might be what's keeping fat locked away in your belly, bum or thighs – and fasting is one way to release it.

FASTING MAINTAINS LEAN MUSCLE

The more muscle you have, the more calories you burn at rest. And before you say you don't want big muscles, another way to put that is: the less muscle you lose as you drop in weight, the less your basal metabolic rate falls as you move toward your goal weight. (Remember, your basal metabolic rate is the rate at which you burn calories, so it's really important in order to make staying in shape easier in the long term.) Besides, muscle takes up less room than fat. So, a person with good lean muscle mass will take a smaller dress size or use a narrower belt notch than someone who doesn't have it.

Fasting is better than plain old calorie restriction when it comes to maintaining lean body mass. This is largely because fasting triggers the release of growth hormone (GH), which encourages your body to look for other fuel sources instead of attacking its muscle stores. This is thought to be a survival advantage – back when humans were hunter gatherers it wouldn't have made sense for our muscle mass to reduce when food was scarce – we needed strong legs and arms to hunt down our dinner!

In one study carried out by researchers at Intermountain Medical Center in the USA, participants were asked to fast for 24 hours. During this time, GH levels rose by a whopping 1,300 percent in women and 2,000 percent in men.

Many other studies have investigated the effects of fasting on GH. Like other hormones, GH levels rise and fall throughout the day and night. They tend to be highest at the beginning of a good night's sleep, when our stomachs are empty but our bodies are hard at work repairing in preparation for a new day. Larger or more frequent bursts of GH are released when we continue to fast and also when we take part in vigorous exercise.

GH acts by sending a signal to our fat cells to release some of their contents into the bloodstream. This enables us to use more fat for fuel, instead of burning mainly carbohydrates for energy. GH is also thought to maintain concentrations of another hormone, insulin-like growth factor (IGF-1), which helps our muscles to build more protein.

This is totally different to what happens when you simply cut calories without changing how often you eat. When you hear people saying you should eat little and often to maintain your blood glucose levels, what they're telling you to do, in actual fact, is to avoid this state. This is because whenever you top up your blood glucose levels through eating, your body releases insulin to compensate, and GH levels never get a boost when insulin is around.

It's important to note that more isn't necessarily better when it comes to GH – what's key is resetting the balance between GH release (which happens in the fasted state) and insulin release (which happens in the fed state, however small your meal) in order to stimulate fat loss without losing lean muscle. You never need to fear growing giant muscles as a result of fasting – GH is released in waves and goes back to normal levels quickly as soon as your body has released enough fat to burn.

As mentioned earlier, if you're already slim, it's especially important not to overdo it when fasting. Research published in the academic journal Obesity Research shows that within just two days of complete fasting, there's a dramatic increase in the use of muscle for fuel in people who are already a healthy weight. This is because they have less fat available to burn overall. Perhaps the advice for people who are already svelte but who want to fast for health benefits is to fast little and often rather than to eat little and often.

FASTING PATTERNS GIVE YOU ENERGY WHEN YOU NEED IT

Alongside maintaining your muscle mass to reduce the dip in your metabolic rate that happens as you lose weight, fasting may help with stubborn weight in other ways.

There's a theory that the reduction in calorie burn typically seen after following a calorie-restricted diet may be related more to changes in activity level than to basal metabolic rate. When you're only eating, say, 1,200 calories day after day, it may be difficult to maintain the energy levels and motivation to exercise. But following an intermittent fasting pattern means that you can concentrate your workouts around the times when you're eating. More energy means a tougher workout – and more calorie burn overall.

COMMON QUESTIONS AND ANSWERS

Q   Isn't "not eating" dangerous?

A   It's very important to establish that fasting is not starvation, which, of course, is dangerous. What I'm talking about is the health benefits of increasing the gaps between meals or eating less from time to time.

Some people who are fully signed up to the merry-go-round of traditional dieting will argue that not eating is likely to induce a low-blood-sugar or "hypo" episode. Feeling faint, clammy and unable to concentrate are typical symptoms, happily offset by a visit to the vending machine or, for the health- aware, a snack such as an oatcake or nuts and seeds. I'm not suggesting that snacking should be outlawed – most of the time, I'm more than happy to tuck right in. But fasting challenges the assertion that we can't survive, or even thrive, without five mini-meals a day.

I accept that challenging the blood-sugar story isn't going to win me any popularity prizes. However, the reality of what science is telling us today is that there's no medical consensus on the concept of low blood sugar. The vast majority of us are perfectly capable of regulating our blood glucose level and, although we may feel ravenous between meals, going without food for a few hours won't cause the blood glucose to plummet and, even if it does, our self-preserving mechanisms will kick into action long before we pass out. What this means is that insulin's countermeasure, glucagon, will kick in, releasing those locked-up glucose stores into the blood and bringing the glucose level back within its normal range.

A few words of warning, though… Diabetic "hypos" are a different thing altogether, of course, and can be very dangerous, but they are drug- induced. For people diagnosed as diabetic but who are not yet on insulin medication, fasting has proved promising. In a year-long study on intermittent fasting, the group who fasted every other day stayed off diabetes medication for significantly longer.

Q   Won't I feel light-headed and really hungry on a fast?

A   You might be worried that your blood sugar levels will dip too low between meals and that you'll feel faint and weak. But when you're not eating, other hormonal signals trigger your body to release glucose or make more. In one Swedish study by researchers at the Karolinska Institute, students who'd reported that they were sensitive to hypoglycemia (low blood sugar) felt irritable and shaky during a 24-hour fast, but there was actually no difference in their blood sugar levels – it may all have been in their minds.

It's true that your brain requires about 500 calories a day to keep the grey matter ticking over effectively. The brain's preferred fuel is glucose, which your liver stores around 400 calories-worth of at a time. In a longer fast, the body is forced to increase its production of ketone bodies, which act as a glucose-substitute for your brain. But in the short term, so long as you eat well before and after your fasting period, your body is perfectly able to produce enough glucose to keep your brain happy.

Q   Hang on a minute… My trainer told me that six small meals will fire up my metabolism and stop me feeling peckish. Who's right?

A This is one of those fitness and nutrition "truths" that has been repeated so many times, people are convinced that it's a fact. In one small study at the US National Institute on Aging, researchers found that people who ate only one meal a day did tend to feel hungrier than those who ate three. But beyond eating three meals a day, meal frequency doesn't seem to make a difference to hunger or appetite, so it comes down to what's actually easiest for you. A study published by the International Journal of Obesity showed that people who are overweight tend to snack more often.

Q   Can fasting change my shape?

A   For many women, that last bit of surplus weight is carried around the hips and thighs and it simply won't shift. To solve this problem, I suggest looking to the true body professionals.

According to noted intermittent-fasting expert Martin Berkhan, there's a good reason for this. All the cells in our body have "holes" in them known as receptors. To switch activity on and off in those cells, hormones or enzymes enter the receptors. Fat cells contain two types of receptor – beta 2 receptors, which are good at triggering fat burning, and alpha 2 receptors, which aren't. Guess which is mostly found in the fat stores of your lower body? Yes, our hips and thighs have nine times more alpha 2 receptors than beta.

Q   What about belly fat?

A   All over the Internet you'll see promises that you can get rid of belly fat in a matter of days by taking supplements. We all know that this is simply not true. Stubborn fat around the middle is linked to a number of factors – including stress, alcohol, lack of exercise and a diet high in refined carbohydrates.

Every time you eat something sweet or a refined carbohydrate such as biscuits or white bread, your blood sugar levels rise quickly, causing your pancreas to release the fat-storing hormone, insulin. If you spend the day going from sugary snack to sugary snack, and especially if you wash everything down with a couple of glasses of wine, your body ends up storing more of the calories you eat and you end up with that dreaded "muffin top"!

Stress + refined carbohydrates + alcohol = a recipe for belly fat, especially if you're unlucky enough to be genetically predisposed to weight gain around the middle.

Q   How does fasting help torch belly fat?

A   To burn belly fat, free fatty acids must first be released from your fat cells (this is called lipolysis) and moved into your bloodstream, then transferred into the mitochondria of muscle or organ cells, to be burned (a process known as beta-oxidation).

Glucagon (another pancreatic hormone that has pretty much an equal and opposite effect to insulin) rises around four to five hours after eating, once all the digested nutrients from your last meal have been stored or used up. The purpose of glucagon is to maintain a steady supply of glucose to the brain and red blood cells, which it achieves by breaking down stored carbohydrates and leftover protein fragments in the liver. It also activates hormone-sensitive lipase, which triggers the release of fat from the fat cells, allowing other cells to be fueled by fat as opposed to glucose.

When you're fasting, belly fat can be turned into energy to keep your organs working effectively and, for example, to provide power to the muscles that hold you upright, as well as fueling muscle movement.

In contrast, when you're constantly grazing, your body doesn't need to release glucagon. Instead, the pancreas pumps out insulin, which also acts to maintain blood glucose levels within a narrow range. Insulin encourages the fat cells to keep their fat tightly locked up. Not only that, but any spare glucose that isn't required for energy and cannot be stored can actually be converted into fat.

Q   What else can I do to help get rid of belly fat?

A   Endurance exercise selectively reduces abdominal fat and aids maintenance of lean body mass, so it's great to do in combination with intermittent fasting. Choose a fasting method that will enable you to take regular exercise – gentle activity such as walking will help, but high-intensity training is even better.

Also, a very small recent study, carried out at the University of Oklahoma in the USA, found that quality protein intake was inversely associated with belly fat, so make sure you fuel up on lean proteins (which your fasting plans are rich in), when you are eating.

Q   What about losing that last 4.5kg (10lb)?

A   This is often the hardest weight to shift. Not only that, it tends to creep back over a matter of weeks after you've finally reached your target weight. A familiar story is the strict diet we follow to get into beach-body shape in time for a holiday: in all the years I've helped people to lose weight, I've lost count of the number of times I've heard people telling me that all their hard work was undone by two weeks of sun, sea and sangria!

Remember that losing weight is all about creating a calorie deficit. Here, fasting is acting in two different ways. First, fasting helps maintain calorie burn – so in theory you can eat more overall and still lose weight. Second, fasting might just be easier to stick to than a boring calorie-counting diet. And when it comes to beach bodies, remember that old saying "a change is as good as a rest". If you're bored of the approach you've taken to weight loss up to now, a short blast of fasting can help you achieve your goal weight without damaging your metabolism.

FASTING AND CANCER

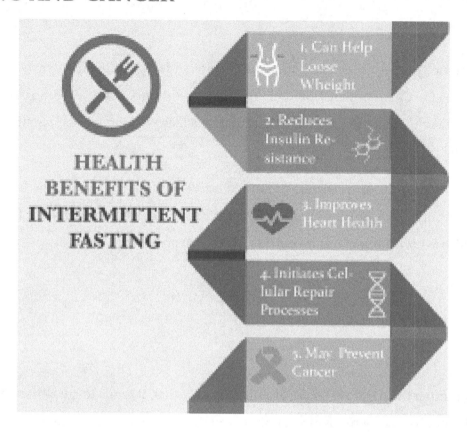

Fasting is considered to be an alternative or complementary treatment for cancer in certain sectors of complementary medicine, and has been popularized by a naturopathic doctor called Max Gerson. However, my focus is not on fasting as a stand-alone treatment but rather on exciting evidence about fasting in cancer prevention and the encouraging results from trials involving fasting during cancer treatment, particularly chemotherapy.

There's evidence that intermittent fasting, and calorie restriction more generally, fights the growth and spread of cancer cells in animals. Often when we read about research on animals, it seems so compelling that we want to see if the same thing will work for us. However, research is so much less likely to be done on humans as, rightly or wrongly, ethics committees are often reluctant to approve the same types of study that are done on animals. As discussed above, in experiments on laboratory animals, diets with 25 percent fewer calories have shown a positive link with longer, healthier life spans. So far there's little empirical study evidence to show the same effect in humans, yet anecdotal evidence is growing that restricting calories, and fasting, activates cell-protecting mechanisms. Research is also underway to find out whether alternate-day fasting can help reduce the risk of breast cancer.

In studies on mice with cancer, fasting appears to improve survival rates after chemotherapy. Hearing of the effects of these animal studies by Valter Longo, ten cancer patients took it upon themselves to try fasting before chemotherapy. The results were published in the medical journal Aging. Of these ten, the majority experienced fewer side-effects as a result of fasting than those eating normally, and the authors concluded that fasting for two to five days before chemotherapy treatment appeared to be safe. This work has yet to be taken to a truly meaningful empirical testing on humans, but it's understandable that cancer patients are excited by the potential of calorie restriction and fasting, not least by it helping the body to mitigate the effects of cancer treatment and specifically chemotherapy.

DETOXING

Personally, I no longer like the word "detox". It's been used and abused by marketeers in their quest to sell, sell, sell fancy products, when, in fact, detoxing is something that the body does naturally every hour of the day. However, until someone comes up with a better word, "detox" will have to do.

HOW WE BECOME TOXIC

A toxin is anything that has a detrimental effect on cell function or structure. Toxins are materials that our bodies cannot process efficiently. Over time they build up and, as a result, our systems function below par, leaving us drained, tired and frequently ill. People become "toxic" in many ways – through diet, lifestyle and the environment, as a natural by-product of metabolism, and through genetic lineage. Stress and harmful emotions can also create a kind of toxic environment.

Toxins include, but are not limited to:

- Food additives, flavorings and colorings.

- Household and personal cleaning chemicals, which are both inhaled and absorbed via the skin.

- Agricultural chemicals, such as pesticides, fungicides and herbicides.

- Heavy metals, which occur naturally but are poisonous.

- Oestrogens, which enter the environment due to human usage of the contraceptive pill and HRT.

- Xeno-oestrogens, which are chemicals that mimic oestrogen.

…And here are the most common ways people become toxic on the inside:

- Eating a poor diet. This includes low-fiber foods, fried foods and foods tainted with synthetic chemicals. Unlike live foods (fresh fruits and vegetables), these lack the enzymes that assist proper digestion and assimilation, and the fiber or bulk that assists proper elimination. They're also void of essential vitamins, minerals and other basic nutrients.

• Eating too much. Over-eating puts a great amount of stress on our digestive system. The body must produce hydrochloric acid, pancreatic enzymes, bile and other digestive factors to process a meal. When we over-eat, the digestive system finds it hard to meet the demands placed upon it. The stomach bloats as the digestive system goes into turmoil. Foods aren't broken down properly and tend to lodge in the lower intestine. Vital nutrients are then not absorbed.

• Inadequate water intake. When the body isn't receiving enough water, toxins tend to stagnate, hindering all digestive and eliminative processes.

• Exposure to synthetic chemicals in food and environmental pollutants. A clean, strong system can metabolize and excrete many pollutants, but when the body is weak or constipated, they're stored as unusable substances. As more and different chemicals enter the body, they tend to interact with those already there, forming second-generation chemicals that can be far more harmful than the originals.

• Being stressed. Stress hinders proper digestion, absorption and elimination of foods.

• Overuse of antibiotics. Antibiotics have a damaging effect on the intestines, especially if they're taken for extensive periods of time. Reducing the use of unnecessary antibiotics will also help minimize the very real danger of bacterial resistance.

• Lack of exercise. This lowers metabolic efficiency, and without circulatory stimulation, the body's natural cleansing systems are weakened.

• Eating late at night. The human body uses sleep to repair, rebuild and restore itself. In essence, the body uses the sleeping hours to cleanse and build. When a person goes to sleep with a full stomach, the body isn't at rest but is busy digesting and processing food. In addition, the body requires gravity to assist the passage of food from the stomach down the digestive tract.

Q   If the body detoxes itself anyway, why bother to do anything further?

A   Just as your home or office can become dusty and dirty, so your body can become clogged up with toxins and waste matter from the environment. A healthy body is able to disarm toxins by breaking them down, storing them in fat tissue or excreting them. However, here's the crux – many, if not most, people are depleted in the nutrients needed to detox optimally, and chronic health problems, sluggishness and weight gain are common results.

If you've never given your digestion much thought, don't beat yourself up about being neglectful. Unlike the head or the tips of the fingers, the gut contains very few nerve endings. What this means is, we're not so aware when things aren't working well. When you have a headache, you feel every throbbing pulse and do something about it. In contrast, gut problems go unresolved and uncared for over long periods.

The good news is, when you improve digestion, a whole range of seemingly unrelated health issues can improve. For example, it's not only the job of the white blood cells (the leukocytes) to defend your body since the digestive system forms the basis of your immune system with the action of beneficial bacteria. Improving the ecology of the gut can be achieved with a juice fast and healthy diet.

USING A JUICE FAST TO DETOX

A juice fast stands head and shoulders above other fasting techniques in its self-healing effect and is often mentioned in the context of detoxing the body.

Juice fasting is based on consuming juices and broths only, whereas intermittent fasting adds lean protein and fat for the feeling of fullness. Studies have shown that eating as little as 10g (¼oz) of essential amino acids (found in high-quality proteins) can switch off autophagy. Therefore, a juice fast is best placed to give your body a good "spring clean" because juices are typically very low in protein.

The simple act of juicing a fruit or vegetable will help you absorb more of the nutrients from it. The caveat here is that you should make the juice fresh rather than drink pasteurized fruit juice from a carton or bottle. The process of juicing eliminates a lot of the fiber that needs to be digested. Cutting out the bulk and drinking only the juice means that you can very effectively hit your antioxidant targets in one small cup. Juice provides tiny "particles" of nutrients that are readily absorbed into the bloodstream.

Fresh juices provide a highly effective fast-track and – importantly – easy delivery mechanism for the body to absorb and process key vitamins, minerals and plant chemicals (phytonutrients) that are so beneficial to our health. A fresh juice contains a concentration of nutrients that have been separated from pulp, making it easier to consume what's required to assist the healing process. In essence, a fresh juice should be considered more of a body tonic than a tasty drink.

Q Will I get withdrawal symptoms on a juice fast?

A The folklore of fasting is littered with stories about the dramatic side-effects of a juice fast. This is usually because the contrast between the diet and lifestyle before and after is simply too great. Or, in some cases, the enterprising individual has decided to "retox", that is go on an almighty bender before entering detox – not a good idea.

One of the most dramatic side-effects I ever witnessed was when a client was coming off a 20-year-long diet cola habit during a juice-fasting retreat. Her symptoms were akin to what you'd expect from coming off a class-A drug. The rest of the detox group watched mesmerized at her descent from bubbly, bouncy guest on arrival to a sweating, vomiting, pale-faced shadow of her former self after just 24 hours of juicing. Even I was a little worried. Luckily, her troubled time was followed by a rapid and dramatic improvement two days later, at which point she declared that she felt "reborn" and would never touch a drop of cola again.

So, learn from my diet cola story and start with a transition diet. Fasting can be a challenge physically and psychologically. I recommend having at least three days on the Countdown Plan to prepare. Juice fasting should be undertaken for between one and five days for optimum results – usually once or twice a year. Any longer requires more management and should only be considered when there are adequate reserves (body fat) or if there's a specific medical condition. Some people find that weekend-long juice fasts four times a year are helpful.

Q What are the most common side-effects of a juice fast?

A   Let me be frank – a juice fast isn't a good idea for a romantic break or naughty weekend away. During a juice fast the capacity of the eliminative organs – lungs, liver, kidneys, and skin – is greatly increased, and masses of accumulated metabolic wastes and toxins are quickly expelled. It's like pressing the accelerator button on your body's waste disposal unit. As part of the eliminative process, your body will be cleansing itself of old, accumulated wastes and toxins. This typically throws up symptoms such as offensive breath, dark urine, increased faecal waste, skin eruptions, perspiration and increased mucus. As I said, it's not exactly romantic!

Your digestive system is the star of a fasting program. Poor digestion can be a hidden cause of weight gain, or more accurately, water retention. For example, if your body's responding to an allergy or intolerance, it will often retain water. So, when fasting, there's often a "quick-win" water loss that equates to an extra kilo being lost.

Q   What about fiber?

A   The process of juicing extracts the pulp (fiber) of the fruits and vegetables so on a juice fast it's a good idea to restore some bulk to maintain a healthy transit of waste matter through the gastrointestinal tract. Psyllium husks, a soluble form of fiber, do just the trick as, when taken with adequate amounts of fluids, they absorb water to form a large mass. In people with constipation, this mass stimulates the bowel to move, whereas in people with diarrhea it can slow things down and reduce bowel movements.

Some recent research also shows that psyllium husks may lower cholesterol. It's thought that the fiber stimulates the conversion of cholesterol into bile acid and increases bile acid excretion. In addition, psyllium husks may even decrease the intestinal absorption of cholesterol.

Psyllium comes from the plant Plantago ovata and is native to India. It is readily available in health food shops and online stores, either as husks or in powdered form. In non-fasting, normal dietary conditions, whole grains provide dietary fiber and similar beneficial effects to psyllium, so a supplement isn't needed unless recommended by your health care practitioner.

Q   Can colon cleansing help?

A   Your bowels are not just "poo pipes". Toxins and metabolic wastes from the blood and tissues are discharged into the intestinal canal to be excreted from the body. Not surprisingly, one of the long-established techniques to support the body's elimination organs during a fast is colon hydrotherapy or enemas. This is a technique that involves taking in water into the large intestine, also known as the bowel, to assist the removal of waste.

Colon hydrotherapy is not a new procedure. Enemas and rituals involving the washing of the colon with water have been used since pagan times. The first recorded mention of colon cleansing is on an Egyptian medical papyrus dated as early as 1500BCE. Ancient and modern tribes in the Amazon, Central Africa and remote parts of Asia have used river water for bowel cleansing, usually as part of magic-medical rites of passage performed by priests or shamans. Colon-cleansing therapies were an important part of Taoist training regimens and these therapies still form one of the fundamental practices of yoga teaching. Hippocrates, Galen and Paracelsus, who are recognized as the founding fathers of Western medicine, described, practiced and prescribed the use of enemas for colon cleansing. In Europe and the USA, colon-cleansing treatments were popular in the early decades of the 20th century and were often performed on patients by doctors practicing in sanatoria (health spas) and hospitals. From the 1920s to the 1960s, most medical practitioners were in favor of regular enemas, and these were often used as part of hospital treatment.

PART 3

REJUVENATION

FASTING AND MOTIVATION

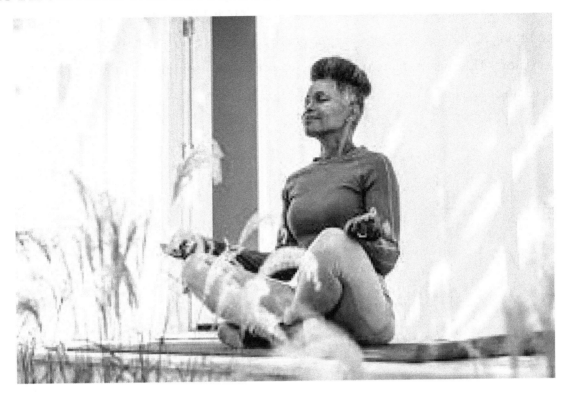

The final motivator, when thinking about incorporating fasting with exercise, is that it could give you more energy to train. There are lots of arguments over whether diet or exercise is more important when it comes to losing weight.

You may be familiar with the saying "you can't out-train a bad diet". While it's probably true that exercise alone isn't going to get you the body you want if you pay no attention to what you eat, dieting without exercise isn't a good idea either. After all, exercise comes with an impressive array of health benefits itself from heart and lung health, to stress relief, to maintaining strong bones.

When it comes to muscle strength and the way you look, exercise is the clear winner over diet. Researchers at Ann Arbor University in Michigan looked at how women's bodies responded to diet alone versus exercise alone. They found that, as expected, diet was more effective at reducing body weight, but exercise was more effective when it came to losing fat and maintaining muscle.

The thing is, getting the motivation to exercise can be hard when you're "on a diet" because you're always eating less than you're burning off and you often feel like you just don't have the energy. The good thing about fasting is that the gaps between meals are longer so when you do eat, you get to eat more. This means that you can time your exercise around the times when you've eaten and are feeling energetic. You're more likely to work harder!

MEDITATION

For those with ambition above and beyond the physical benefits of fasting, getting into the fasting state of mind can be helped by meditation, and if you have the time and inclination at least once in your life, a week's retreat can take the fasting experience to another level.

Meditation can be viewed in scientific terms for its effects on the mind and the body. During meditation, a marked increase in blood flow slows heart rate, and high blood pressure drops to within normal ranges. Recent research indicates that meditation can also boost the immune system and reduce free radicals – in effect, a slowing down of the ageing process.

There's much talk about the power of meditation and how you can use your mind to manifest great piles of money. But, becoming more aware of your mind is not just about manipulating it or attempting only to have positive thoughts – rather, it's about the ability to direct your attention toward or away from the mind at will.

My most intensive fast was on a 10-day silent meditation retreat during my time in India. One evening, five days into the experience when I was seriously doubting my judgement about freezing my butt off in a cold cave in the Himalayas, I had what I've come to realize was a "breakthrough" moment. In spiritual terms I'd describe it as a moment of grace. With a raw, pure energy of infinite magnitude, my mind flashed through formative experiences – good and bad – that had shaped my life. As my mind was swept along on this emotional rollercoaster, my body conveniently left the room, leaving me nowhere to run or hide… or at least that was how it felt!

Even more strangely (and I realize I may lose a few of you here!), during this experience it felt like my spine had dissolved to be replaced by a light-filled serpent. I was left astounded, uplifted and more than a little confused. Given that I was in the middle of a silent retreat, I couldn't even talk to anyone about what I had experienced.

It felt like all the vertebrae in my spine had dissolved at once, to be replaced with an energy much like an electric current. Even more bizarre was the fact that this energy surge was joined by an unshakable vision of a cobra-like snake replacing my spinal column.

Seeking answers, the day I left the meditation retreat I went straight to an Internet café. Within a few minutes I'd discovered that Hindu mythology describes the "serpent power" that lies coiled at the base of the spine as a kind of universal energy. Reportedly, this energy is awakened in deep meditation or enlightenment.

However, let me offer a word of caution before your expectations are set on a one-way ticket to nirvana. If, like many of us, you're the kind of person who never switches off, who even on holiday has the day scheduled from dawn till dusk, the mind experience that can accompany fasting may pass you by altogether. If you want to know yourself better, fasting in a gentle, supportive and quiet environment can help you accomplish a gentle re-boot both physically and mentally, and possibly a little spiritually too. Fasting needs some willpower in the beginning and patience as you move forward. Creating the right environment to enter the fasting state of mind, both inside and outside the body, is really helpful.

When I first started to meditate, I tried too hard. Furiously studying the science of the mind or contorting your face into Zen-like expressions won't work. The only way to experience meditation is actually to experience it. It can be maddening. You'll be trying to meditate for hours and then, just when you're ready to give up, you might get a flash of something akin to what you were aiming for. Yet, in that momentary shift you might see how you could choose to do a few things differently, or how some really small things have a huge impact on you, and how easy it would be to make a few minor changes. Many great thinkers have talked about breakthroughs and inspiration. The most famous of all was probably Albert Einstein, who said that no problem can be solved from the same level of consciousness that created it.

So, if you do manage to get your mind to stop its usual chatter through meditation, try asking yourself a question when all is calm. For example, if you always react to something uncomfortable by quashing the emotion with food, then meditation can create a gap to ask why. Sometimes there's a clear answer to that question, and sometimes there isn't. Usually, it takes a bit of time.

YOGA

Yoga is often lumped together with meditation since the kind of person who likes yoga is often into meditation, and vice versa. For people with a poor attention span, yoga can be a good way of getting into a calm state without the need ever to sit cross-legged.

There are many forms of yoga and it's a case of having a go and seeing which suits you best. Regardless of which tradition you choose, good yoga teachers can make you walk out of the class feeling a foot taller and ready to take on the world. My advice would be:

- If you're gentle by nature, try Hatha.

- If you're into precision and detail, go for Iyengar.

- If you like the spiritual side of yoga, opt for Sivananda.

- If you want yoga to help you sleep, try Yin.

- If you're fit and physical, Ashtanga or Vinyasa "flow" yoga will be more your bag.

- If you really want to sweat, try Bikram, or "hot yoga". It's not for the faint hearted and has some medical contra-indications, but it's considered seriously addictive by devotees.

SELF-CONTROL

If you're into popular psychology or consider yourself a "Tiger Mum" (or Dad), you might well have come across the famous longitudinal "Stanford University Marshmallow Study", first started in the 1960s by Stanford psychology researcher Michael Mischel. The purpose of the original experiment was to find out at what age children develop the ability to wait for something they really want, and subsequent studies over many years tracked the effects of deferred gratification on a person's future success. Mischel's experiment went like this:

NUTRITIONAL RULES FOR FASTING

EAT WELL

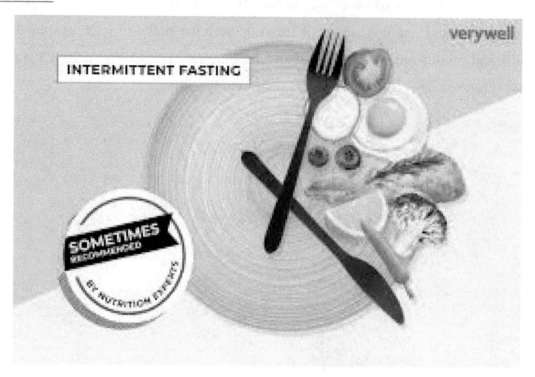

The problem with most fasting information is that it only focuses on the fasting bit, not on what you need to eat. If you're eating fewer calories, what you do eat becomes even more important. Why? We need nutrients for the glands and organs of the body to thrive and burn fat. Restricting nutrients by living on processed foods can deprive the body of the essential vitamins, minerals, fats and proteins it needs to maintain a healthy immune system, recover from injury or illness, keep muscles strong and maintain the metabolism. That's why this book includes these nutrition rules and practical fasting plans and recipes to help guide you.

RULE 1: ONLY EAT "REAL" FOOD

This means no fake food and no diet-drinks. If you grew up in the UK, chances are you'll have fond memories of bright orange corn snacks and fizzy drinks that turned your tongue red or blue. It's to be hoped that now you're "all grown up 'n' stuff", you eat lots of rocket and Parmesan salads, roasted artichoke and monkfish. If only that was the case for all of us. Celebrity chefs may make out that this is the norm but it just isn't. Most people still eat a diet full of processed, refined, low-fiber, nutrient-deficient foods.

Not all processed food is bad, though. In fact, some of it's great. Canned food without added sugar or salt and freshly-frozen fruit and veg are just a couple of examples of stellar staples for your larder. It's the low-calorie, low-fat, oh-so-easy snacks and meals that you need to watch out for since they're often loaded with chemicals and hidden sugars.

In many low-fat products the fat is simply replaced by processed carbohydrates in the form of sugar. Read the label of your regular low-fat treats (apart from dairy products where low fat is fine) and I'll bet you'll see words ending with "-ose". Various forms of sugar, be it sucrose, maltose, glucose, fructose, or the vaguely healthy-sounding corn syrup, are all bad news for weight gain, especially around the middle.

Heavily processed foods can also be high in chemicals. There's a real and present danger that chemicals in the environment may have a blocking effect on hormones that control weight loss. When the brain is affected by toxins, it's possible that hormone signaling is impaired. The reason why we're unsure as to the extent of the problem is that it's impossible to test for the thousands of chemicals that are contributing to the "cocktail" effect on the body. Err on the side of caution and control what you can. Keep foods "real"!

But what makes up a real-food diet?

PROTEIN

Protein is made up of amino acids, often called the "building blocks of life", and we need all of them to stay alive and thrive. Proteins from animal sources – meat, dairy, fish and eggs – contain all the amino acids and are therefore classed as "complete" proteins. Soya beans also fall into this category. Once and for all, eggs are healthy. Eggs have had a tough time of it over the years. First the salmonella scare, then the unfair link to cholesterol. Eggs are low in saturated fat and if you eat eggs in the morning, you're less likely to feel hungry later in the day.

Vegetable sources provide incomplete proteins. If you're vegetarian or vegan, you'll get your protein from nuts, seeds, legumes and grains but you need a good variety of these to ensure that you get the full range of essential amino acids.

TOP TIP:

• Include more beans and lentils in your meals. Examples include kidney beans, butter beans, chickpeas or red and green lentils. They're rich in protein and contain complex carbohydrates, which provide slow and sustained energy release. They also contain fiber, which may help to control your blood fats. Try adding them to stews, casseroles, soups and salads.

CARBOHYDRATES

Carbs are one of the most controversial topics in nutrition and weight loss. For years we've been told that we eat too much fat, and that saturated fat is the main cause of heart disease. But recently, some experts have challenged this view, suggesting that carbohydrate is responsible for the obesity epidemic and a whole host of diseases. Should we cut carbs, avoid fat or simply reduce our food intake and exercise more?

When the body is starved of carbohydrates it looks for energy in its glycogen stores. Water binds to every gram of glycogen so it's easy to get dramatic weight loss – the only problem is that it's mostly water weight! Along with those glycogen stores you'll begin to lose fat but not at a rate higher than a healthier (and easier) weight-loss method.

The truth is there are healthy fats and healthy carbohydrates. Avoiding carbs altogether is unnecessary and potentially dangerous. The key is in recognizing that not all carbs are created equal. Low glycemic index (GI) carbohydrates, found in fiber-rich fruits, beans, unrefined grains and vegetables, are important for good health and can actively support weight loss – for example, through reducing appetite and energy intake.

However, high-GI refined carbohydrates, such as those found in soft drinks, white bread, pastries, certain breakfast cereals and sweeteners, not only make it harder to lose weight but could damage long-term health. Studies show that eating a lot of high-GI carbohydrates can increase the risk of heart disease and Type-2 diabetes.

TOP TIP:

•   Eat bulky carbs to become slim. When you choose "big" foods like fruits, vegetables, salads and soups, which are bulked up by fiber and water, you're eating a lot of food that fills you up, but not a lot of calories.

FAT

Since fat is the greatest source of calories, eating less of it can help you to lose weight. However, fat is actually a vital nutrient and is an important part of your diet because it supplies the essential fatty acids needed for vitamin absorption, healthy skin, growth and the regulation of bodily functions. In fact, eating too little fat can actually cause a number of health problems.

The right kinds of fat, in the right amounts, can also help you to feel fuller for longer, so try not to think of fat as your mortal diet enemy, but rather a useful ally in the pursuit of your healthier lifestyle! Adding a little fat to your meals helps your body absorb nutrients and enhances the flavor of your food, so recipes have been created with this in mind. Choose monounsaturated fats or oils (e.g., olive oil and rapeseed oil) as these types of fats are better for your heart. Coconut oil can be a good choice for cooking as it's heat-stable.

TOP TIPS:

•   Increase essential fats – aim for at least two portions of oily fish a week. Examples include mackerel, sardines, salmon and pilchards. Oily fish contains a type of polyunsaturated fat called omega 3, which helps protect against heart disease. If you don't eat fish, use flaxseed oil in salad dressing and snack on walnuts.

- If you use butter, stick to a thin scraping on bread and just a smidgen for flavor in cooking.

- Choose lean meat and fish as low-fat alternatives to fatty meats.

- Choose lower-fat dairy foods such as skimmed or semi-skimmed milk and reduced-fat natural yogurt.

- Grill, poach, steam or oven bake instead of frying or cooking with oil or other fats.

- Watch out for creamy sauces and dressings – swap them for tomato-based sauces. Add herbs, lemon, spices and garlic to reduced-fat meals to boost flavor.

- Use cheese as a topping, not a meal – in other words, no macaroni cheese! Choose cheese with a strong flavor, such as Parmesan or goat's cheese so that you only need to use a small amount.

RULE 2: CUT OUT SUGAR

Too much sugar makes you fat and has an ageing effect on the skin. Sugar links with collagen and elastin and reduces the elasticity of the skin, making you look older than your years. The recipes I provide use low-sugar fruits to add a little sweetness – and the occasional drizzle of a natural sweetener such as honey is fine – but, in general, sugar is bad news and best avoided.

TOP TIP:

• Stick to dark chocolate if you need a chocolate "fix" (which simply is the case sometimes!), as most people need less of it to feel satisfied.

RULE 3: WATCH THE ALCOHOL

Over the years the alcohol content of most drinks has gone up. A drink can now have more units than you think. A small glass of wine (175ml/5½fl cup) could be as much as two units. Remember, alcohol contains empty calories so think about cutting back further if you're trying to lose weight. That's a maximum of two units of alcohol per day for a woman and three units per day for a man. For example, a single pub measure (25ml/¾fl oz) of spirit is about one unit, and a half pint of lager, ale, bitter or cider is one to one-and-a-half units.

TOP TIP:

• If you're out for the evening, try out some healthy soft drinks such as tonic with cordial, or an alcohol-free grape juice as a tasty substitute to wine. Alcohol-free beers are also becoming increasingly popular and are available in most pubs and bars.

RULE 4: EAT FRUIT, DON'T DRINK IT

If you consume around 1 liter (35fl oz/4 cups) fruit juice, remember you'll be imbibing 500 calories. That's fine if you're juice fasting, but too much if it's simply a snack. You could tuck into a baked potato with tuna and two pieces of fruit for the same number of calories.

TOP TIPS:

• Choose herbal teas (especially green tea, which may aid fat loss).

• Feel free to have a cup or two of tea or coffee. A small amount of milk is allowed but keep it to a splash when you're fasting.

• Sip water throughout the fast, aiming for a fluid intake of around 1.2–2 liters (40–70fl oz/4¾–8 cups) a day. This will not only help to keep hunger pangs at bay, it will also keep you hydrated.

RULE 5: AVOID THE PITFALLS

TOP TIPS:

•　　Top up before you fast. When you first start fasting, you may feel hungry during the times when you'd normally have a meal and you may also feel slightly light-headed if you have sugary foods as your last meal. This isn't a sign that you're wasting away or entering starvation mode, and these feelings of hunger will usually subside once that usual meal time has passed. Try to get your carbohydrate intake from fruit, vegetables and whole grains and eat a good amount of protein, which will fill you up for longer. Following the fasting plans will make this as straightforward as possible.

•　　Stock up for quick meals. Make sure you always have ingredients in your fridge and cupboards for meals that can be put together quickly, such as stir- fries, soups and salads.

•　　Don't polish off the kids' plates. Eating the children's leftovers is a fast track to weight gain for parents. Put the plates straight into the sink or dishwasher when the children have finished their meal, so you won't be tempted!

•　　Downsize your dinner plate. Much of our hunger and satiation is psychological. If we see a huge plate only half full, we'll feel like we haven't eaten enough. But if the plate is small but completely filled, we'll subconsciously feel that we have eaten enough.

•　　Beware of the Frappuccino effect. Black coffee only contains about 10 calories but a milky coffee can contain anything from 100 calories for a standard small cappuccino to a whopping 350+ calories for a Grande with all the trimmings. Much like the plate size, shrink your cup size and shrink your waist line. Don't be afraid to ask for half the milk – spell it out: "Don't fill up the cup." I do it all the time and the best baristas get it right first time!

•　　The sandwich has become the ubiquitous carb-laden "lunch on the go". Lose the top piece of bread to cut your refined carbohydrates and instead fill up with a small bag of green salad leaves and healthy dressing.

• Don't try to change everything at once. Bad habits are hard enough to break as it is. Focus on breaking one at a time.

• If you're a parent, choose your meal skipping wisely. I've tried fasting with a toddler who doesn't understand why Mummy isn't eating and will, quite literally, shove a fistful of tuna pasta into my mouth.

• Get the portions right. If you're restricting the number of meals you're having, it makes sense that the portion sizes need to be bigger than they would be if you were eating five mini-meals a day. Use the recipe section as a guide to how big your portions should be.

PART 4

ANTI-AGING EXERCISES

FITNESS RULES FOR FASTING

WHY EXERCISE?

That old adage, "Daily exercise maketh for a healthy life and lively mind", is all well and good, but the saboteurs of all good intentions, Temptation, Procrastination and Distraction, tend to make exercise an erratic achievement for most people.

Exercise is especially challenging if you're juggling the demands of parenthood. Even though I know I'll feel much better afterwards, some days if my husband didn't proverbially kick me out of the door with my running togs on, I myself would most likely fall victim to the three scourges. Whether it's the long-drawn-out bedtime rituals of frisky toddlers or the clearing up of spaghetti-smeared kitchen walls, parenting saps desire to do anything at all in the evening other than collapse on the sofa with a glass of wine in hand to watch the latest Scandinavian import TV series. Or maybe that's just me.

But really, do we have to exercise? It's a question I'm often asked on retreat. Many people think that exercise is just about burning off calories, but there's so much more to it than that. Along with helping you to achieve and maintain your ideal weight, physical activity can do the following:

- Reduce your risk of heart disease, stroke, type-2 diabetes and some cancers.

- Help keep your bones strong and healthy.

- Improve your mood, reduce feelings of stress and help you sleep better.

- Give you strength and flexibility – attributes that seem to translate as much mentally as they do physically.

I also believe that on top of all these worthy benefits, exercise adds life to your years.

Sometimes it's a simple matter of making exercise more important to you. Also, if you're paying up front for an exercise class, you may find it's harder to miss. My days are dramatically improved by 30–60 minutes of exercise, whether it's running with my dog on the beach or Pilates with the girls. Exercise provides variety, buzz, a glow, a sense of achievement and perspective, plus it helps offset any guilt about enjoying that glass of Sauvignon at the end of the day!

HOW MUCH EXERCISE DO YOU NEED?

In 2010 the World Health Organization (WHO) issued global recommendations on the amount of physical activity we need to stay healthy. They recommend that adults (aged 18–64) should build up to at least 2½ hours of moderate intensity aerobic activity, 1¼ hours of vigorous intensity activity, or a combination of the two each week. We should also incorporate two sessions of muscle-strengthening activities, such as weight training, every week. Although we can meet these recommendations by doing just five 30-minute workouts a week, less than a third of British women are active enough for health. And the benefits don't stop at 30 minutes. WHO stresses that additional benefits can be achieved if we double these minimum recommendations.

Focus is often placed on structured physical activity, such as hitting the treadmill or a spin class, but this is far from being the only factor when it comes to the calorie-burn equation. We've all heard the advice about getting off the bus a stop early, or taking the stairs instead of the lift, but in reality, how useful is this? Well, just think about it... as technology progresses we're at our computers for longer and longer periods each day, we shop online rather than going to the high street, we catch up with friends over Skype or Facebook rather than meeting them in the flesh, we watch TV to relax at the end of a busy day and sometimes we're just so busy that we don't think we can allow ourselves an extra five minutes to walk rather than take the car... the thing is, if you're looking to lose weight, the total energy you burn off has to be higher than the amount you eat and every little step helps.

Collectively, unstructured activities are referred to as non-exercise activity thermogenesis (NEAT) and include all activity-related energy expenditure that's not purposeful exercise. NEAT is actually pretty cool since some of us actually alter NEAT levels according to what we eat without even thinking about it. In other words, one of the secrets of the naturally slim is that they fidget and move more if they over-eat. In fact, one of the ways I was taught to help identify different body types during my training in India was to notice how much of a fidget people were when I was consulting with them! Without fail, those who had "ants in their pants" were the naturally slender types. So, if you're more of a couch potato, walking off dinner is clearly a very good idea! A basic pedometer can track how far you walk each day, and trying to

beat yesterday's step count can be addictive. The next generation of activity monitors track every move you make, and some even help you to understand your sleep patterns.

WHAT COUNTS AS EXERCISE?

Physical activity doesn't just mean sweating it out at the gym – any movement that gets you slightly out of breath, feeling warm and a little bit sweaty, and that makes your heart beat faster, counts (yes, I know what you're thinking and that kind of workout counts too). You can choose from sport, active travel, structured exercise or housework. Even small changes are beneficial and you'll get more benefit from a brisk walk every day than from dusting off your gym membership card once a month. If you've never been very active, it's not too late to start. The key to developing an active lifestyle that you can keep up long term is to find an activity you enjoy.

FINDING INSPIRATION

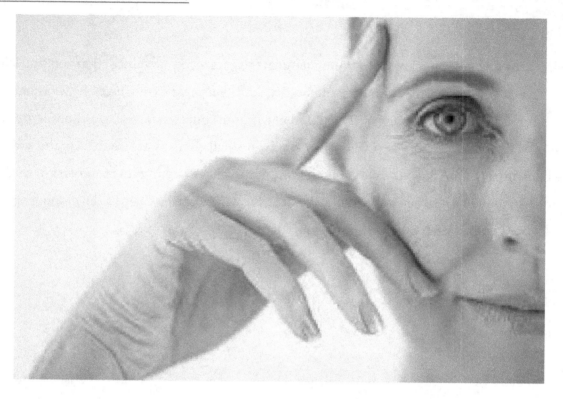

I've found that nothing works better than a bit of inspiration when it comes to changing habits. Over the last two decades, charity events such as marathons, 10km runs, cycle sportive and adventure racing have helped to motivate people to train with a goal in mind. Who would have thought that tens of thousands of women wearing sparkly bras would happily do the "Moonwalk" through the night in London and Edinburgh, kept going only by a sense of camaraderie and a shared purpose to raise money for breast cancer research?

Gyms, too, have revolutionized – it's no longer just about feeling the burn. Classes such as Zumba®, salsa and hula hooping, where having a laugh is every bit as important as burning off calories, have become part of many people's fitness regimes. "Outdoor gyms", like those run by military fitness types, have got all shapes, sizes and ages into the mud and pushing out the press-ups of a Sunday morning. For those willing to go even further, road-or mountain-biking, kitesurfing and triathlon provide accessible competitive events that you can now do much more easily at your own level.

TOP TIPS:

- Book an active holiday to get yourself started.

- Sign up for a charity run or hike.

- Achieve inner calm with yoga or sweat it out in a Bikram studio.

- If dancing's your thing, try Sh'Bam™, the latest craze to follow Zumba®.

- If you have kids, encourage them to play active games and join in too.

- Work off job frustrations with a boxing or martial arts class.

- Treat yourself to a one-to-one with a personal trainer.

- Volunteer for a local conservation project or do some heavy-duty gardening.

- Get back to what you were good at in school – badminton and netball are popular team sports that stand the test of time.

- Improve your commute to work by walking or cycling.

SIMPLE RULES FOR EXERCISE

RULE 1: TAKE THE FIRST STEP

As the saying goes, "Every journey starts with a single step". If there's anything preventing you from taking that first step, take some time to think about how you can overcome this. From there, set yourself a realistic activity goal for the week. Make sure you write it down and, even better, tell a loved one that you're thinking/going to do it – it makes it more real to share your conviction.

RULE 2: TAKE IT FURTHER

The next step is to monitor your progress – an activity diary is an ideal way to do this – and plan to add a little more each week. Keep setting new goals and challenging yourself. Variety is also vital as you can get into a rut with your exercise program just like with anything else. Follow the lead of international sport coaches who insist on variety to keep minds fresh and stimulated, or sign up to a sport where you'll be under the watchful gaze of a coach.

RULE 3: TAKE CARE

If you're new to exercise, or haven't done any for some time, you should always check with your doctor before starting a new exercise program. The benefits of activity almost always outweigh the risks, but if you have a health

condition or are just starting out, your doctor will be able to advise on any activities that you should avoid or take extra care with.

RULE 4: GO FOR THE BURN

You'll get the best benefits from a structured exercise plan, especially if you do some of your training at a high intensity and include some weights. But if you're not quite ready for that, fitting extra movement into your day is a good way to get started. If you take the stairs instead of the lift, get off the bus or train one stop early and are generally more active without actually working out, you could lose at least 6kg (1st) in 12 months, so long as you don't eat more to compensate! If you're already exercising regularly, instead of just focusing on doing more exercise, take every opportunity to do things the active way.

When you're fasting, a great way to boost your calorie burn is to focus on increasing your NEAT. Together with the advice below on exercising, this will make sure you're doing everything you can to achieve the best shape possible.

ACTIVITY	TIME NEEDED (MINUTES)
1. Skipping	8
2. Jogging	12
3. Gardening (weeding)	14
4. Swimming (leisurely pace)	14
5. Cycling (light effort)	14
6. Scrubbing the floor (vigorous effort)	15
7. Vacuuming	18
8. Dancing	19
9. Playing with children	21
10. Walking the dog	24
11. Food shopping (at the supermarket)	28
12. Driving a car	32
13. Computer work	43

You might be disheartened when the running-or step-machine tells you you've burnt 87 calories when you've been sweating for at least 15 minutes. After all, it

doesn't even add up to a skinny cappuccino. Don't despair! You burn fat even after exercise because you primarily use carbohydrate fuel during the exercise, which takes time to replace, so in the meantime, your body burns fat for energy. In other words, your metabolism is raised for a little while after your workout.

EXERCISING AND FASTING

The obvious second part to the puzzle is exercise. Exercise has many wonderful benefits. It can help with depression and anxiety, while also helping you to attain your aesthetic goals. Exercise is also going to play a part in the balancing of the hormones mentioned earlier. Exercise promotes the production of HGH, but will also help drain glycogen stores quickly.

What is the best exercise when fasting?

It is popular belief that long drawn-out cardio at a steady pace is the best way to burn fat. In my experience, this is not the case. Although it has its benefits, when it comes to burning fat and the IF lifestyle, I've had far more success with HITT training for both female and male clients.

High Intensity Interval Training (HITT)

If burning fat is your mission, I recommend HITT training. Fast paced workouts that can be done in 30 minutes make this ideal for someone with a busy lifestyle. HITT can be done with bodyweight exercises, barbells, kettlebells and dumbbells. I usually look to use exercises that use more than one muscle group. For example, a row rather than a bicep curl. The name of the game is short bursts at near maximum effort. Below are some guidelines you can play with. They are meant as guidelines, not gospel!

➤ 20 second exercise – 10 second rest (Advanced)

➤ 10 second exercise – 20 second rest (Intermediate)

➤ 10 second exercise – 30 second rest (Beginner)

Rounds:

➤ 8+ (Advanced)

➤ 3-6 (Intermediate)

➤ 1-3 (Beginner)

Number of exercises:

➤ 7+ (Advanced)

➤ 5-6 (Intermediate)

➤ 3-5 (Beginner)

Example workouts

Beginner

➤ Squat

➤ Running on the spot

➢   Star Jumps

Intermediate

➢   Burpees

➢   Weighted squat

➢   Press Up

➢   Medicine Ball Slam

➢   Battle Ropes

Advanced

➢   Burpee/ High Jump

➢   Box Jump

➢   Kettlebell Swing

➢   Clean & Press

➢   Battle Ropes

➢   Kettlebell Row

EXERCISE AND THE 16/8 FAST

THE 16:8 DIET

	DAY 1	DAY 2	DAY 3	DAY 4	DAY 5	DAY 6	DAY 7
MIDNIGHT / 4 AM / 8 AM	FAST	FAST	FAST	FAST	FAST	FAST	FAST
12 PM	First meal	First meal	First meal	First meal	First meal	First meal	First meal
4 PM	Last meal by 8PM	Last meal by 8PM	Last meal by 8PM	Last meal by 8PM	Last meal by 8PM	Last meal by 8PM	Last meal by 8PM
8 PM / MIDNIGHT	FAST	FAST	FAST	FAST	FAST	FAST	FAST

But what about exercising while fasting? As you'll know from the "Fit You and Your Life to Fasting" chapter, the 16/8 fasting pattern is often used by people who are looking to get into their best shape ever, and workouts are usually done in a fasted state.

However, it's important to remember that most of the studies on exercise while fasted were done on men, and we know that women's bodies may respond differently. This means that, when it comes to the 16/8 fast, the rules for men and women are slightly different.

EXERCISE AND THE 5/2 FAST

THE 5:2 DIET

DAY 1	DAY 2	DAY 3	DAY 4	DAY 5	DAY 6	DAY 7
Eats normally	Women: 500 calories Men: 600 calories	Eats normally	Eats normally	Women: 500 calories Men: 600 calories	Eats normally	Eats normally

If you're going to do the 5/2 fast, it's best to avoid prolonged or hard exercise on your 500-calorie days. However, it's fine to do this sort of exercise a couple of hours after your first meal the following day. And do make sure that if you're exercising the day before your 500-calorie day, you end the day with a proper meal.

Although you'll be going for periods of the day without food, the fasting plan covers all your nutritional requirements. To ensure that you're getting everything your body needs to fuel an active lifestyle, I encourage you to eat more during your eating "windows" if you feel hungry. Keep healthy snacks to hand so that you're not tempted by junk food if hunger pangs strike.

Recovery, Rest & The Importance of Sleep

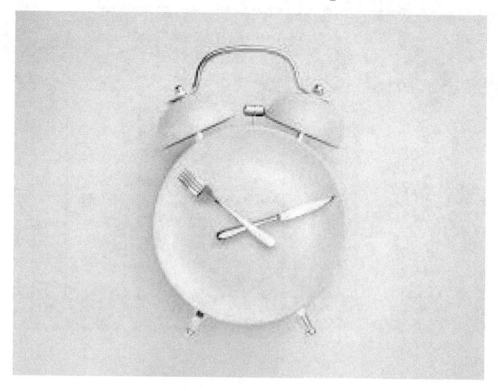

As promised, here is the third (perhaps most important) part of the weight loss puzzle which is often neglected. Sleep! Getting proper sleep can skyrocket your results - here's how.

Our body primarily enters an anabolic (building) type phase during sleep. Our body goes to work repairing damage, replacing cells, and believe it or not, burning fat. Shawn Stevenson explains this in his book "Sleep Smarter:

21 Essential Strategies to Sleep Your Way to A Better Body Better Health and Bigger Success". This book has outlined key hormones you should know about for weight loss, but there are many more. Some help initiate repair and growth and some help keep us awake and/or alert. One of the big factors dictating the creation and release of these hormones is quality sleep. Stevenson cites studies showing sleep deprivation can be linked to high levels of hormones such as cortisol and insulin (Remember what too much insulin does?). He also mentions hormones correlated with fat burning that are only secreted during sleep and darkness. Remember how HGH helps burn fat? Quality

sleep is linked to the creation of this hormone. If you're not getting quality sleep at the right times, all the exercise and healthy eating may not yield the results you were hoping for. If you've ever dieted before while thrashing yourself in the gym only to see little to no results, you know how frustrating this is! Perhaps proper sleep was the missing piece you needed!

4 tips to sleep better at night

TIP 1 – Get more sun

Our body's circadian system or "body clock" plays a huge role in the production of hormones. This is heavily influenced by sunlight. Stevenson explained Light, specifically morning sunlight, signals your glands and organs it's time to wake up, queuing them to produce day time hormones (most of these helping keep you alert and awake). If our bodies get inefficient sunlight in the morning and then too much artificial light at night (such as TV, laptops and smart phones) our circadian clock gets jumbled. This can cause our glands to produce hormones that prevent us sleeping. Lack of quality sleep is going to hinder the production of hormones such as HGH and could even spike the creation of hormones such as insulin. If this happens, we won't burn fat over night!

TIP2 – Avoid screens before bedtime

If you are someone who watches TV until 11pm or falls asleep to YouTube on your phone, the quickest way to improve sleep would be to stop using your devices at least an hour before bedtime. Remember how our body clock is impacted by sunlight? It's also impacted by artificial light. Our eyes are a major light sensor and the blue light produced by our favorite screens stimulate our body to produce day time hormones which are primarily for keeping us awake and active. With these bad boys circulating our body, falling asleep will be hard and our body won't produce those sweet anabolic hormones we need to repair and lose weight. Some of which Stevenson cited as only being produced in the dark. Interesting!

NOTE: My clients often argue that watching TV or some other device helps them go to sleep and without it they toss and turn. The information above is to achieve quality sleep and even though you might feel that way, I find in most cases this is simply because the client has made this a habit.

I encourage you to find other activities to replace your device, rather than lying in the dark stressing about not going to sleep.

TIP 3 – Sleep in darkness

Although this might seem apparent after the first two tips, some of my clients neglect this tip when not told. We can't control lights outside, such as street lamps and annoying security lights, but these could still affect our sleep on the molecular level, interrupting repair and leaving us tired the next day. Black out your windows with heavy duty curtains to stop pesky outside lights ruining your healing process!

P.S If it wasn't obvious turn out lamps, nightlights as well.

TIP 4 – Quality not Quantity

One of the most beneficial points I took away from Stevenson's book was that there is a sweet time window during the night where sleep is the most beneficial. During this window, our body produces the best number of hormones needed for repair and fat loss. He explained this was roughly between 10pm and 2am leaving every hour out of this window as a bonus. He also noted this could vary depending on time of year and what time zone you are in but suggested getting to bed as soon as possible after dark falls.

Improving your sleeping habits is key to weight loss, building muscle and living a healthier life in general. This important factor is often neglected in weight loss programs perhaps being the missing piece you needed! Quality sleep is going to ensure proper adaptation of key hormones for fat burning and might even be more important than increasing your exercise in the gym. Set a consistent bed time and make sure to get to bed about 30 to 60 minutes prior.

FASTING SAFELY

By now I hope that you have an open mind to the many benefits of fasting and that you're excited about giving it a go. If you've read this book and are still trying to decide if, when, or how to give fasting a try, remember that you'll only ever truly "get it" by trying it for yourself.

Before you launch headlong into your new fasting lifestyle, here are a few words of caution. Although fasting has been around for millennia, the science on how and when to fast is in its early stages. For example, there's very little research on how fasting affects fertility.

There are some people who should avoid fasting completely, some who should seek medical advice first, and some situations where it might not be right for you. Fasting isn't something that you should just jump into, and it doesn't suit everyone.

WHEN NOT TO FAST

You should avoid fasting if any of the following apply:

- You are pregnant, breastfeeding, or actively trying for a baby (it's okay to fast if you're getting your body ready to conceive, but please don't consider fasting if there's any chance you could already be pregnant).

- You have ever experienced an eating disorder.

- You are underweight

You should seek medical advice first if any of the following apply:

- You have a long-term medical condition such as cancer, diabetes, ulcerative colitis, epilepsy, anemia, liver, kidney or lung disease.

- You have a condition that affects your immune system.

- You are on medication, particularly medicines that control your blood sugar, blood pressure or blood lipids (cholesterol).

POSSIBLE SIDE-EFFECTS AND HOW TO MANAGE THEM

As we learnt earlier in the book, fasting may make you feel a bit "yucky" at first. Many juice fasters experience headaches through caffeine withdrawal, and feeling hungry is natural when you first try a fast. These effects don't usually last long, and most people find that they're outweighed by the positive effects of fasting.

More serious side-effects may include:

- Dehydration or over-hydration.

- Feeling dizzy or light-headed.

- Extreme fatigue.

- Constipation.

- Nausea or vomiting.

- Insomnia.

- Irregular periods.

Always err on the side of caution and stop the fast if you don't feel well. You can minimize the risk of some side-effects by approaching the fast safely.

END NOTE

I invite you to think of your goals as a journey. This book as the start, and your goal as the finish. The roads and paths in between will vary, and be full of both victories and losses. Your humble beginning and your eventual triumph mean nothing without the winding roads that link them, and vice versa. Everyone admires those who have "made it". Whether that is in regard to weight loss or some other human want like riches or fame. We are especially motivated by those who appear to have come from nothing or succeeded against all odds, but the road that links these two paradigms is just as important as the factors themselves. The roads are scarcely revered unless the end is reached, otherwise it is simply a road leading nowhere, a lost cause

– failure. Those who have nothing or are underprivileged are seldom celebrated unless they manage to follow a path with a successful ending. Your health and fitness journey are not exempt from such parameters. You have most likely started a hundred times. You have most likely trodden many paths seeking your goal, only to find fleeting success or failure. I hope this book will arm you with enough hope to start once again and lead you on the right path to your ultimate victory, perhaps inspiring those around you to take action and do the same.

The Healthy Keto Meal Prep Cookbook with Pictures

Bend the Rules to Lose Weight Tasting Tens of Easy-to-Prep Ketogenic Recipes On a Budget

By

Casey Black

Table of Contents

Introduction

Few aspects are as well known in nutrition research as the tremendous health advantages of low-carb and ketogenic diets. Not only can these diets increase the cholesterol, blood pressure and blood sugar, but they also reduce your appetite, promote weight control and decrease the triglycerides.

A ketogenic diet may be an interesting way to manage such disorders and could accelerate weight loss. Yet it is challenging to follow, because it may be high on red meat and other oily, dried, and salty foods that are notoriously unhealthy. We still may not know anything about the long-term consequences, presumably because it's too hard to stay with that people can't eat this way for a long time. It is also important to note that "yo-yo diets" that contribute to rapid weight loss fluctuation are correlated with increased mortality. Instead of joining in the next common diet that will last just a few weeks or months (for most people that requires a ketogenic diet), strive to accept progress that is manageable over the long term. A healthy, unprocessed diet, abundant in very colorful fruits and vegetables, lean meats, seafood, whole grains, almonds, peas, olive oil, and plenty of water seems to provide the strongest evidence for a long, healthier, vibrant existence.

If you're interested to improve your fitness, this diet book might be worth considering.

Chapter 1: Keto Diet

The ketogenic (keto) diet is commonly known for having a diet (low crab), where the body creates ketones in the liver to be used as energy. It's alluded to by several different names – ketogenic diet, low carb diet, low carb high fat (LCHF), etc. When you consume something rich in carbohydrates, the body can release glucose and insulin.

Glucose is the simplest molecule for the body to transform and use as energy such that it can be preferred over some other energy source.

Insulin is created to process the glucose in your bloodstream by taking it across the body.

The glucose is being used as primary energy; the fats are not required and are thus processed. Usually, on a regular, higher carbohydrate diet, the body can use glucose as the key energy source. By lowering the consumption of carbohydrates, the body is induced into a condition known as ketosis. Ketosis, a normal mechanism the body initiates to help us live while food consumption is limited. During this state, we create ketones, which are formed by the oxidation of fats in the liver.

The ultimate aim of a well-controlled keto diet is to push your body into this physiological condition. We don't do this by deprivation of calories or starvation of carbohydrates.

What Do I Eat on a Keto Diet?

To initiate a keto diet, you may want to prepare accordingly. That implies getting a viable diet plan ready a. What you consume depends on how quickly you choose to get into a ketogenic condition, i.e., ketosis. The further stringent you are on your carbohydrates (less than 25g net carbs a day), the sooner you can reach ketosis.

You want to keep your carbs limited, come more from fruits, nuts, and dairy. Don't consume some processed grains such as wheat (bread, pasta, and cereals), starch (potatoes, beans, legumes) or berries. The small exceptions to this are banana, star fruit, and berries which may be eaten in moderation.

Do Not Eat

Grains: grain, maize, cereal, rice, etc.

Sugar: honey, maple syrup, agave, etc.

Fruit: bananas, grapes, strawberries, etc.

Tubers: yams, potatoes, etc.

Do Eat

Meats: fish, meat, lamb, chickens, chickens, etc.

Leafy Greens: lettuce, cabbage, etc.

Vegetables: broccoli, cauliflower, etc.

Low Fat Dairy: strong cheeses, high-fat milk, butter, etc.

Nuts and seeds: macadamias, walnuts, sunflower seeds, etc.

Avocado and berries – raspberries, blackberries, and other low glycemic

Sweeteners: stevia, erythritol, monk berries, and other low-carb sweeteners

Other fats: palm oil, high-fat salad dressing, fatty fats, etc.

Benefits of a Ketogenic Diet

Several advantages come from being on keto: from weight reduction and improved energy levels to medicinal uses. Mostly, everyone can easily profit from consuming a low-carb, high-fat diet. Below, you'll find a concise list of the advantages you may get from a ketogenic diet.

Weight Loss

The ketogenic diet actually utilizes your body fat as an energy source – but there are clear weight-loss advantages. On keto, your insulin (the fat-storing hormone) level drops greatly and transforms your body into a fat-burning process. Scientifically, the ketogenic diet has demonstrated better outcomes relative to low-fat and high-carb diets, also in the long run.

Control Blood Sugar

Keto reduces blood sugar levels due to the kinds of diet you consume. Studies also suggest that the ketogenic diet is a more efficient way to treat and avoid diabetes relative to low-calorie diets.

If you're pre-diabetic or have Type II diabetes, you should strongly try a ketogenic diet. We have several readers who have had experience in their blood sugar management on keto.

Mental Focus

Many people use the ketogenic diet primarily for improved mental output. Ketones are a perfect source of food for the brain. When you reduce carb consumption, you stop major increases in blood sugar. Together, which will help in increased attention and concentration? Studies suggest that an improved consumption of fatty acids may have affecting benefits to our brain's function.

Increased Energy & Normalized Hunger

By providing your body a stronger and more stable energy supply, you can feel more energized throughout the day. Fats are the most powerful molecule to burn as heat. On top of that, fat is inherently more rewarding and ends up keeping us in a satiated ("full") condition for longer.

Types of Ketogenic Diets

Many people wonder whether carbs are required to grow muscle. Actually, they're not. If you're asking this question, I will presume you know how you accumulate mass.

Your glycogen reserves will also be refilled while on a ketogenic diet. A keto diet is an effective way to grow muscle, but protein consumption is essential here. It's proposed that if you are trying to grow muscle, you could be getting in between 1.0 – 1.2g protein per lean pound of body mass. Putting muscle on can be slower on a ketogenic diet, but that's because the overall body fat is not growing as much.

If, for any reason, you need to add on body fat, too, you will accomplish your targets by various forms of a Ketogenic Diet. There are:

Standard Ketogenic Diet (SKD): This is the classic keto diet that everybody understands and does.

Targeted Ketogenic Diet (TKD): This variant is where you consume SKD but ingest a limited amount of fast-digesting carbohydrates before a workout.

Cyclical Ketogenic Diet (CKD): This variant of keto for bodybuilders and contests goers, usually offering one day a week to carb up and resupplies glycogen stocks.

Common Side Effects of a Keto Diet

Here are some of the more popular side effects that one comes across when people first initiate keto. Frequently the problems contribute to dehydration or loss of micronutrients (vitamins) in the body. Be sure that you're consuming enough water (close to a gallon a day) and enjoying foods containing healthy sources of micronutrients.

Cramps

Cramps (and, more importantly, leg cramps) are a fairly normal occurrence before beginning a ketogenic diet. It's typically happening in the morning or at night, but overall, it's a fairly small concern. It's a warning that there's a shortage of minerals, especially magnesium, in the body. Be sure you consume lots of fluid and eat salt on your meal. Using so will help reduce the lack of magnesium and get rid of the problem.

Constipation

The most frequent source of constipation is dehydration. An easy approach is to maximize water consumption and aim to get as close to a gallon a day as possible.

Trying to make sure veggies have some fiber. Bringing in some high-quality fiber from non-starchy vegetables will fix this issue. Though if that's not enough, normally, psyllium husk powder can work or take a probiotic.

Heart Palpitations

When switching to keto, you may find that the heart is beating both faster and slower. It's fairly normal, so don't think about it. If the condition remains, make sure that you're consuming enough liquids and eating enough salt. Usually, this is adequate to get rid of the issue right away. Though if the problem continues, it might be worth having a potassium supplement once a day.

Reduced Physical Performance

You can have some restrictions on your results when you start a keto diet, but it's generally only from your body transitioning to using fat, when your body changes in utilizing fat for energy, all of your power and stamina will return to normal. If you still notice issues with results, you can see benefits from taking carbs before exercising (or cycling carbs).

Saving Money and Budgeting

A popular myth is that the ketogenic diet is more costly than most diets out there. And, though it can be a little bit more costly than eating grain-stuffed goods, it's still better than many people believe. A ketogenic diet can be more costly than a regular American diet, but it's no different than most clean eating lifestyles. That said, there are always several ways to save money when cooking keto. The key strategies to raise money are the same as in all other budgeting:

Look for offers. There's still a discount or an offer to be had on keto-friendly products out there. Usually, you can find substantial discounts in magazines and newspapers that are delivered to your home, but they can also be paired with in-store specials and manager cuts. As paired, you will save a large portion of your keto groceries.

Bulk purchase and cook. If you're somebody who doesn't want to invest a lot of time in the kitchen, this is the best in all worlds. Buying the food at volume (specifically from wholesalers) will reduce the cost per pound immensely. Plus, you can make ahead food (bulk cook chicken thighs for pre-made beef, or cook whole meals) that are used as leftovers, meaning you waste less time preparing.

Do stuff yourself. Although it's incredibly easy to purchase certain products pre-made or pre-cooked, it still contributes to the price per pound of goods. Try prepping vegetables ahead of time instead of getting pre-cut ones. Try having your stew meat from a chuck roast. Or attempt to produce your mayo and salad dressings at home. The easiest of items will operate to cut back on your overall food shopping.

How to Reach Ketosis

Achieving ketosis is fairly simple, but it may appear complex and overwhelming for all of the details out there. Here's the bottom line about what you need to do, arranged in stages of importance:

Restrict the sugars: Many people prefer to only rely only on net carbohydrates. If you want better outcomes, restrict both. Aim to remain below 20g net carbs and below 35g gross carbs a day.

Restrict the protein consumption: Some people come over to keto from an Atkins diet and don't restrict their protein. Too much protein can contribute to lower levels of ketosis. Ideally, you ought to eat between 0.6g and 0.8g protein per pound of lean body fat. To assist with this, try using the keto calculator >

Stop thinking about fat: Fat is the main source of calories on keto – just be sure you're giving the body plenty of it. You should not lose weight on keto by malnutrition.

Drink water: Aim to drink a gallon of water a day. Make sure that you're hydrating and remaining compliant with the volume of water you consume. It not only helps regulate many important bodily functions, but it also helps manage hunger levels.

Stop snacking: Weight reduction seems to perform well because you have fewer insulin surges during the day. Unnecessary snacking can lead to stalls or delays in development.

Start fasting: Fasting can be a perfect tool to raise ketone levels reliably during the day. There are several different ways to go about it. Add workout in. It's a proven reality that exercise is safer. If you want to get the best out of your ketogenic diet, try putting in 20-30 minutes of workout a day. Also, only a short stroll will help control weight loss and blood sugar levels.

Begin supplementing: Although not normally required, supplementing can aid with a ketogenic diet.

What the Science Tell Us about the Keto Diet

The keto diet has been used to better treat epilepsy, a condition marked by seizures, for more than 100 years. More current trials are investigating the keto diet as an effective nutritional therapy for obesity and diabetes. Clinical results on the effects of the keto diet on these health problems are exceedingly minimal. Studies on the success of the keto diet are performed with limited groups of participants. And, much of the research on Alzheimer's disease depends on testing conducted on experimental animals. To completely evaluate the protection of this eating style, further study is required. Plus, research must be performed on the long-term health implications of the keto diet. Body mass index and human metabolic rates affect how easily various people generate ketones. This suggests that certain individuals lose weight more slowly with the keto diet than others even though they are pursuing the same keto diet schedule. For this community of individuals, the keto diet may be stressful and can affect their enthusiasm for making healthy lifestyle improvements. Plus, many individuals are not willing to continue with the keto diet and gain back weight after adjusting to their former eating style.

Chapter 2: Keto Diet Breakfast Recipes

Keto Hot Chocolate

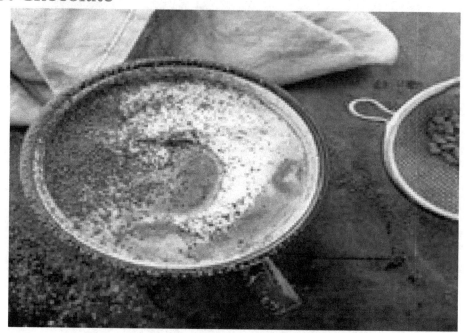

YIELDS: 1

TOTAL TIME: 0 HOURS **20** MINS.

INGREDIENTS

- • 2 Tbsp. of cocoa powder, and more for flavor
- • 2 1/2 Tsp. of sugar keto (diet), (such as swerve)
- • 1 1/4 c. of Water
- • 1/4 c. of heavy cream
- • 1/4 Tsp. of Pure vanilla bean paste
- • Whipped serum, for serving

DIRECTIONS

1. In a small saucepan over medium-low heat, whisk together swerve, cocoa powder or about 2 Tbs. water until smooth and dissolved. Increase heat to medium, add remaining water and cream, and whisk until cook.

2. Mix the chocolate then pour into cup. Serve with whipped cream and a dusting of sugar powder.

Keto Sausage Breakfast Sandwich

YIELDS: 3

TOTAL TIME: 0 HOURS 15 MINS

INGREDIENTS

- 6 large size eggs
- 2 Tbsp. of heavy cream
- Pinch of red chili flakes

- Salt (kosher)
- Finely roasted black pepper
- 1 Tbsp. of butter
- 3 slices of cheddar
- 6 packaged of sausage burgers, cooked as per box directions
- Avocado, sliced

DIRECTIONS

1. Take a small bowl beat eggs, red chili flakes and heavy cream jointly. Season with pepper and salt. Melt the butter in fry pan at low flame. Add around one third of eggs in to pan. Add a piece of cheese in the center or let stay for 1 minute. Roll the ends of egg in to center, filling a cheese. Take out   from heat and continue with leftover egg.

2. Serve eggs in 2 sausage buns with avocado.

Keto Breakfast Cups

YIELDS: 12

TOTAL TIME: 0 HOURS **40** MINS

INGREDIENTS

- 2 Ib. of Pork (ground)
- 1 Tbsp. thyme, finely sliced
- 2 cloves of garlic, finely chopped
- 1/2 Tsp. of Paprika
- 1/2 Tsp. of cumin, ground
- 1 Tsp. of Salt kosher
- Black pepper softly roasted
- 21/2 cup of clean minced spinach
- 1 c. of cheddar, thinly sliced

- Eggs, 12
- 1 Tbsp. of chives that are finely cut

DIRECTIONS

1. 1 Preheat the oven at 400 degrees. Combine the thyme, ground pork, paprika, garlic, salt, and cumin in a large size cup.

2. In each muffin container, add a tiny handful of pork and push up the sides to make a cup. Split the cheese and spinach equally in cups. Break the egg and add the salt and pepper on the top of each cup. Cook for around 25 minutes until the eggs are fixed and the sausage is fried.

3. Garnish and serve with chives.

Best-Ever Cabbage Hash Browns

YIELDS: 2

TOTAL TIME: 0 HOURS **25** MINS

INGREDIENTS

- 2 Large size eggs
- 1/2 Tsp. of garlic, powdered
- 1/2 Tsp. of salt (kosher)
- Freshly roasted black pepper
- 2c. of cabbage that is shredded
- ¼ of small size yellow onions, finely chopped
- 1 Tbsp. of oil (vegetable)

DIRECTIONS

1. Whisk the garlic powder, salt, and eggs together in a large cup. Add black pepper for seasoning. In egg mixture add onion and cabbage and toss to mix properly.

2. Heat oil in a large frying pan. Split the mixture in the pan into 4 patties and   press spatula to soften. Cook until soft and golden, around three minutes on each side.

Chocolate Keto Protein Shake

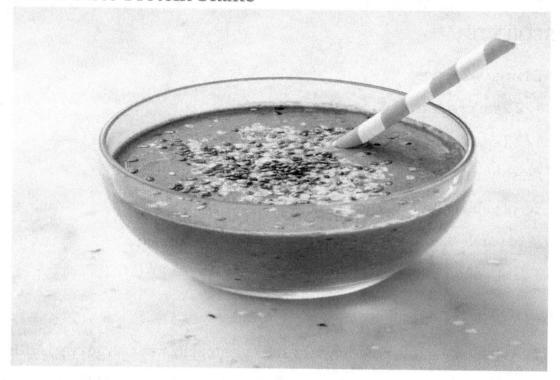

YIELD: 1

TOTAL TIME: 0 HOURS **5** MINS

INGREDIENTS

- 3/4 c of almond milk
- 1/2 c. of ice
- 2 Tbsp. of Butter (almond)
- 2 Tbsp. of (Sugar free) powder of cocoa
- 3 Tbsp. of keto-diet sugar substitute as per taste (such as Swerve)
- 1Tbsp. seeds of chia or more for serving
- 2 Tbsp. seeds of hemp, or more for serving
- 1/2 Tbsp. of pure vanilla (extracted)
- Salt kosher as per taste

DIRECTIONS

1. Merge all of blending mixture and mix untill soft. Put into glass and serve with hemp seed and chia.

Hard Boiled Egg

YIELDS: 1

TOTAL TIME: 0 HOURS **20** MINS

INGREDIENTS

- 12 large size eggs

- Some water

DIRECTIONS

1. Place the eggs in such a wide saucepan and cover them with one inch of ice water. Keep the saucepan on the burner and get it to a boil. Immediately turn off the flame and cover the saucepan. Let settle down for eleven minutes.

2. Take it out from the pan and switch it to ice water. Until serving or peeling, let it cool for 2 minutes.

Paleo Breakfast Stacks

YIELDS: 3

TOTAL TIME: 0 HOURS **30** MINS

INGREDIENTS

- 3 sausage buns for breakfast
- 1 avocado, finely mashed

- Salt (kosher)
- Black pepper freshly roasted
- 3 large size eggs
- Chives, (for serving)
- Hot sauce, if ordered

DIRECTIONS

1. Cook the breakfast sausage as per the box's instructions.
2. Mash the avocado over the sausage for breakfast and season with pepper and salt.
3. Use cooking oil to spray the medium size pan then spray the interior of mason jar cover. Place the mason jar lid in the middle of the pan and crack the interior of an egg. Add pepper or salt and cook until the whites are set for 3 minutes, then remove the cover and begin to cook.
4. Place the egg on top of the avocado puree. Serve with chives and drizzle with your favorite spicy hot sauce.

Ham & Cheese Breakfast Roll-Ups

YIELDS: 2

TOTAL TIME: 0 HOURS **20** MINS

INGREDIENT

- 4 large size eggs
- 1/4 c of milk
- 2 Tbsp. of finely cut chives
- Salt (kosher)
- Black pepper freshly roasted
- 1Tbsp. of butter

- 1c. of cheddar shredded,(Split)
- 4 slices of ham

DIRECTIONS

1. Whisk the milk, chives, and egg together in a medium cup. Add pepper or salt.
2. Melt the butter in a medium pan over low heat. Put 1/2 of the egg mixture in the pan and shift to make a thin layer that covers the whole plan.
3. Cook for two minutes. Add1/2 cup of cheddar or seal again for 2 minutes, before the cheese has melted transfer to plate, and put 2 slices of ham or rolls them. Repeat and cook with the rest of the ingredients.

Cauliflower Toast

YIELDS: 4 - 6

TOTAL TIME: 0 HOURS **45** MINS

INGREDIENTS

- 1 cauliflower (in medium size)
- Large size egg
- 1/2 c. of cheddar cheese (shredded)
- 1Tsp.of garlic(powdered)
- Salt (kosher)
- Black pepper freshly roasted

DIRECTIONS

1. Set the oven at 425 degree temperature and cover the baking sheet with parchment paper. Finely chopped the cauliflower and switch to a large size cup. Set the microwave at high temperature for 8 minutes. Drain with cheesecloth and paper towels just before the mixture is dry.

2. In cauliflower cup, add the cheddar, garlic powder and egg and season with pepper and salt. Mix it until joint

3. Make a cauliflower into bread forms on prepared baking sheet and bake for 18 to 20 minutes until golden.

4. Switch to a plate cover with the appropriate topping, such as fried egg, mashed avocado, tomato, broccoli, and sausage.

Breakfast Bacon and Egg Salad

YIELDS: 4

TOTAL TIME: 0 HOURS **30** MINS

INGREDIENTS

Bacon vinaigrette

- 4 bacon (slices)
- 1 shallot, thinly sliced
- 3 Tbsp. of red wine(vinegar)
- 1 Tsp. of mustard (Dijon)
- 1/4 Tsp. of salt (kosher)
- 1/4 Tsp. of black pepper
- 4 Tbsp. of Oil

Salad

2 small size eggs

1 Spinach (package)

1/4 c. of crumbled feta

1 pt. of tomatoes and cherry

DIRECTIONS

1. In a large fry pan, cook the bacon. Remove the bacon slices and put on a plate and line with towel paper to drain. Implode half of the bacon until the excess fat has drained, then cut the rest of two pieces into large pieces. Set again.

2. Making the vinaigrette: Add the shallot into the pot in which the bacon has been fried, and sauté for around 1 minute over moderate flame until golden brown. Pour the shallots into a small cup and blend with the pepper, salt, red vinegar, and mustard. Whisk in the oil, and then add the crumbled bacon and blending to combine. Set again.

3. In the same pot, fried each egg and cook until the egg white is fixed.

4. Assemble the salad: Combine the feta, lettuce, tomatoes, cherry, spinach and the remaining sliced bacon in a large size dish. Cover with vinaigrette.

5. Place the salad in two cups and cover it with the fried egg. Immediately serve.

Keto Blueberry Muffins

YIELD: 1

TOTAL TIME: 0 HOURS **40** MINS

INGREDIENTS

- 2 1/2 c. of almond Flour

- 1/3 c. of Keto diet sugar (such as Swerve)

- 1 1/2 Tsp. of baking powder

- 1/2 Tsp. of baking soda

- 1/2 Tsp. salt kosher

- 1/3 c. of melted butter

- 1/3 c. of Sugar free almonds milk

- 3 large size eggs

- 1 Tsp. of pure vanilla extract

- 2/3 of c. of fresh blueberries

- ½ of lemon zest (as an option)

DIRECTIONS

1. Preheat oven to 350° and line a 12-cup muffin pan with cupcake liners.

2. In a large bowl, whisk to combine baking powder, baking soda, almond flour, salt kosher and swerve. Whisk in eggs, vanilla, almond milk, melted butter and almond milk until just together.

3. Gently fold lemon zest (if using) and blueberries until uniformly divided. Scoop uniform quantity of butter into every cupcake liner and cook until slightly golden brown and insert a toothpick into the middle of a muffin comes out clean, 23 minutes. Let cool slightly before presenting.

Mason Jar Omelets

YIELDS: 2

TOTAL TIME: 0 HOURS **15** MINS

INGREDIENTS

- Nonstick cooking oil
- 4 large size eggs
- 2/3 c. of cheddar shredded
- ½ of onion, thinly sliced
- 1 Chopped capsicum
- 1/2 c. of ham (sliced)
- Salt kosher
- Freshly roasted black pepper

- 1Tbsp. of Chives that are finely sliced

DIRECTIONS

1. Oil the nonstick baking spray into two liter mason jars.

2. Break two eggs into each jar. Between two jar divide the onion, ham capsicum, and cheese and season with pepper and salt.

3. Put cover on jar and mix until eggs are scrambled and all ingredients are mixed.

4. Remove the cover and place in the oven. Microwave for 4 minutes on low flame, and looking every 30 seconds. Garnish with chives, and serve immediately.

Keto Fat Bombs

YIELDS: 16

TOTAL TIME: 0 HOURS **30** MIN

INGREDIENTS

- 8 oz. of cream cheese, mitigated at room temp.
- 1/2 c. of keto diet (peanuts) butter
- 1/4 c of (coconut oil)
- 1/4 Tsp. of salt (kosher)

- 1/2 c. of dark chocolate (keto diet) (such as Lily's)

DIRECTIONS

1. Cover the baking sheet with a tiny parchment paper. Mix the peanut butter, salt, cream cheese and 1/4 cup of coconut oil in a medium dish. With the help of hand blender beat the mixture for around 2 minutes until all ingredients are properly mixed. Keep the dish for 10 to 15 minutes in the freezer to firm up slightly.

2. Using a tiny cookie spoon or scoop to make a Tbs. sized balls until the (peanut butter) mixture has been settled. Keep in the freezer for 5 minutes to harden.

3. Besides that, making a drizzle of chocolate: mix the cocoa powder and the leftover coconut oil in a safe microwave dish and cook for 30 seconds until completely melt. Drizzle over the balls of peanut butter and put them back in the fridge to harden for 5 minutes.

4. Keep the cover and freeze it for storage purpose.

Cloud Eggs

YIELDS: 4

TOTAL TIME: 0 HOURS **20** MINS

INGREDIENTS

- 8 large size eggs
- 1 c. of Parmesan, thinly sliced
- 1/2 lb. of Ham deli, diced
- Salt (kosher)
- Freshly made black pepper
- For serving, finely sliced chives

DIRECTIONS

1. Heat the oven at 450 °C and spread cooking oil on a large baking sheet. Separate the yolks and egg whites, yolks are keep in small cup and egg whites are keep in large cup egg whites. Use a hand blender or whisk break egg whites before stiff peaks shape and cook for 3 minutes. Fold in the ham and parmesan or season with pepper and salt.

2. Spoon the 8 mounds of egg onto the heated baking dish and indent centers to make nests. Cook for around 3 minutes, until lightly golden.

3. Spoon the egg yolk cautiously into the middle of each nest, then season with pepper or salt. Cook for around 3 minutes more until the yolks are ready.

4. Before presenting, garnish it with chives.

Chapter 3: Keto Diet Lunch Recipes

Cobb Egg Salad

YIELDS: 6

TOTAL TIME: 0 HOURS **20** MINS

INGREDIENTS

- 3 Tbsp. of mayonnaise
- 3 Tbsp. of yogurt
- 2 tbsp. of vinegar with red wine
- Salt (kosher)
- Black pepper freshly roasted
- 8 hard-boiled eggs, sliced into 8 pieces, and more for garnishing.
- 8 bacon strips, fried and crumbled, and more for garnishing.

- 1 avocado, cut finely
- 1/2 c. of blue cheese, crumbled, and more for garnishing
- 1/2 c. of halved cherry tomatoes, and more for garnishing
- 2 Tbsp. of chives that are finely chopped

DIRECTIONS

1. Mix   the yogurt,   red vinegar   and   mayonnaise   together   in   a   small cup. Seasoning with pepper and salt.

2. Mix the avocado, bacon, eggs, pineapple, cherry tomatoes and blue cheese, softly together in a large serving cup. Gently roll in the mayonnaise coating until the all ingredients are finely coated, and then sprinkle with pepper and salt.

3. Serving with chives and supplementary toppings

Taco Stuffed Avocado

YIELDS: 4 - 8

TOTAL TIME: 0 HOURS **25** MINS

INGREDIENTS

- 4 large size avocados
- 1 lime juice
- 1 Tbsp. of olive oil (extra-virgin)
- 1 medium size onion, minced
- 1 lb. minced meat of beef
- 1 taco seasoning pack
- Salt (kosher)
- Blinerack pepper freshly roasted

- 2/3 of c. of chopped Mexican cheese
- 1/2 c. of chopped Lettuce
- 1/2 c. of Grape tomatoes (Sliced)
- Sour milk, for garnishing

DIRECTIONS

1. Pit and halve the avocados halve and pit. Scoop out a bit of avocado with the help of a spoon, forming a wide layer. Dice extracted avocado and later put aside for use. Pinch the lime juice (to avoid frying!) at all the avocados.

2. Heat the oil in a medium size pan over medium heat. Add the onion and roast for around 5 minutes, until soft. Break up the meat with a wooden spatula then add ground beef and taco for seasoning. Sprinkle with pepper and salt, and roast for around 6 minutes until the beef is no more pink. Drain the fat after removing from the heat.

3. Fill up the each avocado halve with meat, then and coat with cheese, reserved avocado, tomato, onion, lettuce, and a dollop of sour cream.

Buffalo Shrimp Lettuce Wraps

YIELDS: 4

TOTAL TIME: 0 HOURS **35** MINS

INGREDIENTS

- 1/4 Tbsp. of butter
- 2 cloves of garlic, chopped
- 1/4 c. of Hot sauce, for example, Frank's
- 1 Tbsp. of olive oil (extra-virgin)
- 1 lbs. of Chopped and finely diced shrimp, tails (cut)
- Salt kosher
- Black pepper freshly roasted
- 1 head Romaine, different leaves, for garnishing
- 1/4 of red onion, finely minced

- 1 rib celery, finely chopped
- 1/2 c. of Crumbled blue cheese

DIRECTIONS

1. Making the buffalo sauce: Melt the butter in a small pan. When fully melted, then add chopped garlic and simmer for 1 minute, until golden brown. Add hot sauce and stir together. Switch the heat to low whilst the shrimp is frying.

2. Making shrimp: Heat oil in a large frying pan. Put some shrimp and sprinkle with pepper and salt. Cook, turning midway, until both sides are opaque and pink, around 2 minutes on each side. Turn off the flame and add the (buffalo) sauce and toss to fill.

3. Prepare wraps: In the middle of the romaine leaf add a little scoop of shrimp, then coat with celery, blue cheese and red onion.

Keto Broccoli Salad

YIELDS: 4

TOTAL TIME: 0 HOURS **35** MINS

INGREDIENTS

For the salad:

- Salt (kosher)
- 3 broccoli heads, sliced into bite-size parts
- 1/2 c. of cheddar shredded
- 1/4 red onion, finely cut
- 1/4 c. of almonds sliced (baked)

- 3 bacon slices, fried and crumbled
- 2 Tbsp. of Chives that are finely cut

For the dressing:

- 2/3 of c. of mayonnaise
- 3 Tbsp. of Vinegar (Apple Cider)
- 1 Tbsp. of Mustard dijon
- salt kosher
- Black pepper freshly roasted

DIRECTIONS

1. Bring the 6 cups of (salted) water to a boil in a medium pot or frying pan. Prepare a big bowl of ice water while waiting for the water to heat.

2. Put some broccoli florets to the boiling water and simmer for 1 to 2 minutes, until soft. Detach with a slotted spoon, and put in the prepared ice water cup. Drain the florets in a colander while it is cold.

3. In a medium dish, whisk together the ingredients for the dressing. Season with pepper and salt to taste.

4. In a large bowl, combine all the salad ingredients and pour over the coating. Toss before the components are coated in the dressing. Refrigerate until prepared

Keto Bacon Sushi

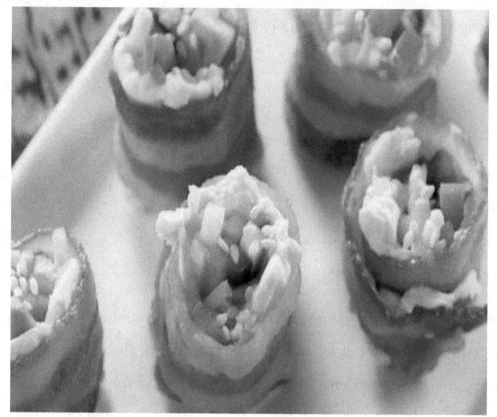

YIELDS: 12

TOTAL TIME: 0 HOURS **30** MINS

INGREDIENTS

- 6 bacon pieces, (halved)

- 2 Persian cucumbers, cut finely

- 2 medium size carrots, cut finely

- 1 avocado, in slices

- 4 oz. of melted cream cheese, (cooked)

DIRECTIONS

1. Preheat oven to 400 ° degrees. Cover a baking sheet and match it with a cooling rack and aluminum foil. Put some bacon pieces in an even layer and cook for 11 to 13 minutes until mildly crisp but still pliable.

2. Mean a while, cut avocado, cucumbers, and broccoli into pieces around the width of bacon.

3. Spread an equal layer of cream cheese on each slice until the bacon is cold enough to touch it. Split up the vegetables between the bacon uniformly and put them on one side. Tightly roll up the vegetables.

4. Serve   and garnish with   sesame seeds.

Keto Burger Fat Bombs

YIELDS: 20

TOTAL TIME: 0 HOURS **30** MINS

INGREDIENTS

- Cooking oil
- 1 lbs. of ground-based meat
- 1/2 Tsp. of Powdered garlic
- Salt Kosher
- Black pepper freshly roasted
- 2 Tbsp. of cold butter,20 (sliced)
- 2 oz. of cheddar cheese 20 (sliced)
- Lettuce berries, meant for garnishing
- For garnishing, finely sliced tomatoes
- Mustard, for garnishing

DIRECTIONS

1. Preheat the oven at 375 °C and oil mini muffin container with cooking oil. And season the beef with garlic powder, salt, and pepper in a medium dish.

2. In the bottom of each muffin tin cup add the 1 Tsp. of beef equally, and fully covering the bottom. Place a layer of butter on top and add 1 Tsp. of beef over the butter to fully cover.

3. In each cup, place a slice of cheddar on top of the meat and place the remaining beef over the cheese to fully cover.

4. Bake for about 15 minutes, before the meat is ready. Let wait until cool.

5. Using a metal offset spoon carefully to release each burger out of the tin. Serve with salad leaves, mustard and onions.

Keto Taco Cups

YIELDS: 1 DOZEN

TOTAL TIME: 0 HOURS **30** MINS

INGREDIENTS

- 2 c. of Cheddar (Sliced) cheese
- 1 Tbsp. of Olive Oil (extra-Virgin)
- 1 small size chopped onion
- 3 cloves of garlic , finely chopped
- 1 lbs. of meat, ground
- 1 Tsp. of chili(in powdered form)
- 1/2 Tsp. of Cumin ,ground

- 1/2 tsp. of Paprika
- Salt (kosher)
- Black pepper freshly roasted
- Sour cream, to serve
- Diced avocado, planned for serving
- Cilantro finely chopped, for serving
- Tomatoes, chopped, for garnishing

DIRECTIONS

1. Preheat the oven to 375 ° and use parchment paper to cover a wide baking sheet. Add 2 teaspoons of cheddar a half inch away. Cook for around 6 minutes, until creamy and the edges begin to turn golden. Leave the baking sheet for a minute until cool.

2. Besides that, apply the oil in the muffin tin bottom with a cooking spray, then carefully pick up the slices of melted cheese and put them on the muffin tin bottom. Add another inverted muffin container until cool for 10 minutes. Using your hands to help shape the cheese around the twisted pan because you do not have a second muffin tin.

3. Preheat the large size pan over medium heat. Put the onion and simmer for around 5 minutes, mixing frequently, until soft. Whisk in the garlic, then add the ground beef to break up the beef with the help of wooden spoon. Cook for around 6 minutes, until the beef is no longer pink, and then drain the fat.

4. Place the meat back in the pan and season with cumin, chili powder, cinnamon, paprika, and pepper.

5. Move the cups of cheese into a serving bowl. Cover it with cooked ground beef and serve with cilantro, sour cream, tomatoes, and avocado.

Copycat Chicken Lettuce Wraps

YIELDS: 4

TOTAL TIME: 0 HOURS **30** MINS

INGREDIENTS

- 3 Tbsp. of Sauce (Hoisin)
- 2 Tbsp. Soy sauce (low-sodium)

- 2 Tbsp. vinegar from rice wine

- 1 Tbsp. of sriracha (as an option)

- 1 Tsp. oil with sesame seeds

- 1 Tbsp. olive oil (extra-virgin)

- 1 medium size chopped onion

- 2 cloves of garlic, chopped

- 1 Tbsp. of freshly coated ginger

- 1 lbs. of Chicken, ground

- 1/2 c. of drained and diced canned water chestnuts

- 2 green onions, cut finely

- Salt kosher

- Black pepper freshly roasted

- Large leafy lettuce for serving (leaves separated),

- Fried white rice, for garnishing(as an option)

DIRECTIONS

1. Making a sauce: Whisk together the soya sauce, the hoisin sauce, the sriracha the rice wine vinegar, the Sriracha and the sesame oil in a tiny cup.

2. Heat the olive oil in a large pan over a medium-high heat. Put some onions and cook for 5 minutes until soft, then stir the garlic and ginger and cook for 1 more minute until golden brown. Add ground chicken and cook until the meat is opaque and mostly finished, trying to break up the meat with a wooden spoon.

3. Add the sauce and simmer again for 1 or 2 minutes, before the sauce is slightly reduced and the chicken is thoroughly cooked. Switch off the flame, add green onions and chestnuts and mix. Season with pepper and salt.

4. Spoon rice and add a big scoop of chicken mixture (about 1/4 cup) into the middle of each lettuce leaf (if used). Instantly serve

Egg Roll Bowls

YIELDS: 4

TOTAL TIME: 0 HOURS **35** MINS

INGREDIENTS

- 1 Tbsp. of oil for vegetables
- 1 clove of garlic, chopped

- 1 Tbsp. fresh ginger chopped
- 1 lbs. of pork, ground
- 1 Tbsp. of oil with sesame seeds
- 1/2 onion, cut finely
- 1 c. of Carrot(sliced)
- 1/4 green, thinly sliced (cabbage)
- 1/4 c. of soya sauce
- 1 Tbsp. of sriracha
- 1 small size green onion, finely chopped
- 1 Tbsp. of sesame seeds

DIRECTIONS

1. Heat the vegetable oil in a large skillet over medium heat. Add the garlic and ginger and roast for 1 to 2 minutes until it is moist. Add pork and roast until there is no more pink color has been shown.

2. Place the pork and add the sesame oil to other side. Add the tomato, cabbage, and potato. Add the soy sauce and Sriracha and whisk to combine with the beef. Cook for 5 to 8 minutes, until the cabbage is soft.

3. Garnish with sesame seeds and green onions and shift the mixture to a serving bowl. Serve immediately.

Caprese Zoodles

YIELDS: 4

TOTAL TIME: 0 HOURS **25** MINS

INGREDIENTS

- 4 large size zucchinis

- 2 Tbsp. of olive oil (extra-virgin)

- Kosher salt

- Black pepper freshly roasted

- 2 c. of cherry tomatoes, sliced in half

- 1 c. of mozzarella cubes, cut into pieces(if large)

- 1/4 c. fresh leaves of basil

- 2 Tbsp. of vinegar (balsamic)

- DIRECTIONS

1. Using a spiralizer, make zoodles with the help of zucchini.

2. In a large cup, add the zoodles mix with the olive oil, and add pepper and salt. Let them marinate for 15 minutes.

3. Add the basil, peppers, and mozzarella in zoodles and toss until mixed.

4. Drizzle and serve with balsamic.

Best-Ever Keto Quesadillas

YIELDS: 4

TOTAL TIME: 0 HOURS **35** MINS

INGREDIENTS

- 1 Tbsp. of olive oil (extra-virgin)

- 1 chopped bell pepper
- 1/2of onion(yellow), chopped
- 1/2 Tsp. of chili powdered
- Salt kosher
- Black pepper freshly roasted
- 3 c. of Monterey jack shredded
- 3 c. of cheddar cheese, shredded
- 4 c. of Chicken shredded
- 1 avocado, cut thinly
- 1 green onion, finely chopped
- Sour cream, for serving

DIRECTIONS

1. Preheat the oven to 400C and cover the parchment paper with two medium size baking sheets.

2. Heat the oil in a medium saucepan over medium heat. Season with salt, chili powder and pepper and add onion and pepper. Cook for 5 minutes, until it is tender. Transfer to a dish.

3. In a medium cup, mix the cheeses together. In the middle of both prepared baking sheets, add 1 1/2 cups of cheese mixture. Spread into an even coat and form the size of a flour tortilla into a circle.

4. Bake the cheeses for 8 to 10 minutes before they are melted and slightly golden along the sides. Add one half of   avocado slices, onion-pepper mixture, shredded chicken and avocado slices. Let it cool slowly, then use the small spoon and parchment paper and carefully fold and lift one end

of the cheese "tortilla" over the end with the topping. Return to the oven to heat for an extra 3 to 4 minutes. To make 2 more quesadillas, repeat the procedure.

5. Split each quesadilla into quarters. Before serving, garnish it with sour cream and green onion.

Cheeseburger Tomatoes

YIELDS: 4

TOTAL TIME: 0 HOURS **20** MINS

INGREDIENTS

- 1 Tbsp. of olive oil (extra-virgin)
- 1 medium size onion, minced

- 2 cloves of garlic, chopped

- 1 lbs. of ground-based meat

- 1 Tbsp. of ketchup

- 1 Tbsp. of mustard (Yellow)

- 4 sliced tomatoes

- Salt kosher

- Black paper freshly roasted

- 2/3 of c. of cheddar shredded

- 1/4 c. of Iceberg lettuce shredded

- 4 coins with pickles

- Seeds of sesame, for garnishing

DIRECTIONS

1. Heat oil in a medium pan over medium heat. Add the onion and cook for approximately 5 minutes until soft, then add the garlic. Add the ground beef, split up the meat with a wooden spoon and roast for around 6 minutes until the beef is no longer pink. Drain fats. Season with pepper and salt, then add the ketchup and mustard.

2. Because they are stem-side out, tossing tomatoes. Cut the tomatoes into six slices and be cautious not to cut the tomatoes full. Fold the slices carefully. Divide the tomatoes equally with the cooked ground beef, then fill it with lettuce and cheese.

3. Add sesame seeds and pickle coins for flavoring.

No-Bread Italian Subs

YIELDS: 6

TOTAL TIME: 0 HOURS **15** MINS

INGREDIENTS

- 1/2 c. of mayonnaise
- 2 Tbsp. of Vinegar with red wine
- 1 Tbsp. olive oil (extra-virgin)
- 1 tiny clove of garlic, finely chopped
- 1 Tsp. of seasoning (Italian)
- 6 slices of ham
- 12 salami sliced

- 12 pepperoni, sliced
- 6 provolone slices
- 1 c. of romaine(chopped)
- 1/2 c. of red peppers (roasted)

DIRECTIONS

1. Making a smooth Italian dressing: whisk the mustard, mayonnaise, garlic, oil, and Italian seasoning together in a small bowl until they are mixed.

2. Prepare the sandwiches: Layer a pieces of pork, two pieces of pepperoni, two pieces of salami and a piece of provolone.

3. In the center, add a handful of Romaine and a few roasted red peppers. Drizzle, with fluffy Italian sauce, then roll up and eat. Continue the procedure with the rest of the ingredients until you have 6 roll-ups.

California Burger Bowls

YIELDS: 4

TOTAL TIME: 0 HOURS 20 MINS

INGREDIENTS

For the dressing:

- 1/2 c. of olive oil (extra-virgin)
- 1/3 c. of vinegar (balsamic)
- 3Tbsp. of mustard dijon
- 2 Tsp. of. honey
- 1 clove of garlic , chopped
- Salt kosher
- Black pepper freshly roasted

For the burger:

- 1 lbs. of grass fed organic ground beef
- 1 Tsp. of Sauce (worcestershire)
- 1/2 tsp. of chili Powdered
- 1/2 tsp. onion Powdered
- Salt kosher
- Black pepper freshly roasted
- 1 packet of butter head lettuce
- 1 medium size red onion, sliced (¼)
- 1 avocado,(in pieces)
- 2 Walmart medium size tomato, thinly sliced

DIRECTIONS

1. Making the dressing: Whisk together the dressing components in a medium dish.

2. Making burgers: Mix beef with chili powder, (Worcestershire) sauce and onion powder in another large bowl. Season with salt and pepper and whisk until blend. Shape into 4 patties.

3. Heat a wide grill pan over medium heat and grill the onions until they are crispy and soft, around 3 minutes on at each end. Remove the grill from the pan and add the burgers. Bake until browned and fried to your taste on all ends, around 4 minutes per end for medium.

4. Assemble: Toss the lettuce with 1/2 of the dressing in a wide bowl and split between 4 bowls. Cover each with a patty of steak, tomatoes, fried onions, slices of 1/4 avocado. Drizzle and serve with the remaining dressing.

Chapter 4: Dinner Recipes

Keto Corned Beef & Cabbage

TOTAL TIME: 5 HOURS 0 MINS

YIELDS: 6

INGREDIENTS:

- 3 to 4 1bs. of corned beef
- Onions, 2 (quartered)
- 4 stalks of, quartered crosswise celery
- 1 pack of pickling spices
- Salt (Kosher)
- Black Pepper
- 1 medium size cabbage (green), sliced into 2 wedges

- carrots (2), sliced and split into 2" part
- 1/2 c. of Dijon mustard
- 2 Tbsp. of (apple cider) vinegar
- 1/4 c. of mayonnaise
- 2 Tbsp. capers, finely sliced, plus 1 tsp. of brine
- 2 Tbsp. of parsley, finely cut

Directions:

1. Place corned beef, onion, celery, and pickling spices into a large pot. Add the water to cover by 2", salt with season or Pepper, and bring to the boil. Medium heat, cover, and Simmer very (tender), 3–3 1/2 hours.

2. In the meantime, whisk Dijon mustard and apple cider vinegar in a small bowl and add salt and pepper. And in another bowl, mix capers, mayo, caper brine, and parsley. Season with salt and pepper

3. Added carrots and cabbage continue cooking for 45 minutes to 1 hour more until cabbage is soft. Remove meat, cabbage, and carrots from the pot. Piece of corned beef and season with a little more pepper and salt.

4. Present with both sauces on the side for soaking.

Keto Fried Chicken:

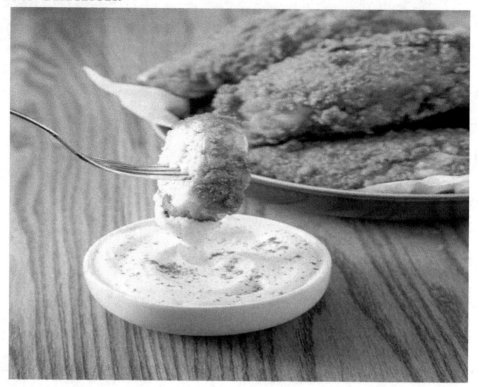

TOTAL TIME: 1 HOUR 15 MINS

YIELDS: 6 - 8

INGREDIENTS

FOR THE CHICKEN

- 6 (Bone-in), chicken breasts with skin, about 4 lbs.
- Salt (Kosher)
- Black Pepper, ground and fresh
- 2 large size eggs
- 1/2 c. of heavy cream
- 3/4 c. of almond flour
- 1 1/2 c. perfectly crushed pork rinds

- 1/2 c. of grated Parmesan, fresh
- 1 Tsp. of Garlic in powder form
- 1/2 Tsp. of paprika

FOR THE SPICY MAYO:

- 1/2 c. of Mayonnaise
- 1 1/2 Tsp. of Hot sauce

DIRECTIONS

1. Preheat oven to 400° and cover a wide baking sheet with parchment paper. Pat dry chicken with paper towels and add salt and pepper.

2. In a small bowl, mix together eggs and heavy cream. In another small dish, mix almond flour, pork rinds, Parmesan, garlic powder, and paprika. Add salt and black pepper.

3. Work at one time, soak the chicken in egg mix, then in the almonds flour mix, pressing to cover. Put the chicken on the lined baking dish.

4. Bake till chicken is gold and internal temp exceeds 165°, about 45 minutes.

5. In the meantime, produce dipping sauce: In a medium dish, mix mayonnaise and hot sauce. Add more hot sauce based on desired spiciness amount.

6. Serve chicken warm with dipping sauce.

Garlic Rosemary Pork Chops:

TOTAL TIME: 0 HOURS 30 MINS

YIELDS: 4

INGREDIENTS:

- 4 pieces of pork loin
- Salt (kosher)
- Black pepper freshly roasted
- 1Tbsp. of Freshly chopped rosemary
- 2 Garlic cloves, minced
- 1/2 c (1 stick) of butter melted

- 1 Tbsp. of Extra-virgin (olive oil)

DIRECTIONS:

1. Preheat the oven to 375 degrees. With salt and black pepper, season the pork chops generously.

2. Mix the honey, rosemary, and garlic together in a shallow dish. Only put back.

3. Heat the olive oil in an oven-safe skillet over (medium-high) heat and add the pork chops. Sear until golden for 4 minutes, flip and bake for a further 4 minutes. Pork chops are appropriately coated with garlic butter for 10-12 minutes.

4. Add more garlic butter to serve.

Keto Bacon Sushi

TOTAL TIME: 0 HOURS 30 MINS

YIELDS: 12

INGREDIENTS:

- 6 bacon strips, cut in half
- 2 cucumbers (Persian), cut thin
- 2 carrots (medium), cut thinly
- 1 (avocado), in slices
- 4 oz. (Creamy) cheese, cooked, soft
- Seeds of sesame (garnish)

DIRECTIONS:

1. Preheat the oven to 400 degrees. Line a baking sheet and match with a (cooling rack) with (aluminum) foil. Lay bacon half with an even surface and cook for 11 to 13 minutes unless mildly crispy but always pliable.

2. In the meantime, split the bacon's size into pieces of cucumbers, broccoli, and avocado.

3. Spread an equal surface of cream cheese from each strip until the bacon is cold enough to touch it. Divide the vegetables into the bacon equally and put them in one hand. Strictly roll up the vegetables.

4. Season with and serve the sesame seeds.

Keto Chicken Parmesan

TOTAL TIME: 0 HOURS 55 MINS

YIELDS: 4

INGREDIENTS:

- 4 boneless without skin breasts of chicken
- Kosher salt
- 1c. of Almond Flour
- 3 big, beaten eggs
- 3 c. of Parmesan, freshly grated, and much more for serving
- 2 Tsp. of Powdered garlic
- 1 1/2 c. of Mozzarella Sliced
- 1 Tsp. of onion in powdered form
- 2 Tsp. of Oregano dried
- Oil for vegetables
- 3/4 c. Sugar-free, low-carb tomato sauce
- Fresh leaves of basil for topping

DIRECTIONS

1. Preheat the oven to 400 degrees. Halve the chicken breasts crosswise with a sharp knife. Season the chicken with salt and pepper on both sides.

2. Put the almond flour and eggs in 2 different shallow cups. Combine the parmesan, garlic (powder), onion (powder), and oregano in the third shallow dish. With salt and pepper, season.

3. Dip the chicken cutlets into the almond flour, then the eggs, the Parmesan mixture, and push to cover.

4. Heat 2 teaspoons of oil in a large skillet. Add chicken and roast, 2 to 3 minutes on each hand, until golden and cooked through. Function as required in batches, inserting more oil as appropriate.

5. Move the fried cutlets to a 9-inch-x-13-inch baking dish, distribute the tomato sauce uniformly over each cutlet, and finish with the mozzarella.

6. Bake for 10 to 12 minutes before the cheese melts. If needed, broil for 3 minutes until the cheese is golden.

7. Until eating, top with basil and more Parmesan.

Tuscan Butter Shrimp

TOTAL TIME: 0 HOURS 55 MINS

YIELDS: 4

INGREDIENTS

- 2 tbsp. of olive oil extra-virgin
- 1 lb. deveined, peeled, lobster and tails cut
- salt (kosher)
- Black pepper freshly roasted
- 3 tbsp. of Butter
- 3 garlic cloves, minced
- 1 1/2 c. of halved tomatoes with cherry
- 3 c. of spinach for kids
- 1/2 c. of heavy cream
- 1/4 c. of Parmesan, finely grated
- 1/4 c. of thinly cut basil
- Lemon wedges meant for serving as an option

DIRECTIONS

1. Heat oil in a frying pan over medium heat. Season the shrimp with salt and pepper all over. Add the shrimp and sear until the underside is golden, around 2 minutes, and then turn until opaque, until the oil is shimmering but still not burning. Remove and set aside from the skillet.

2. Lower the heat to mild and add some butter. When the butter is melted, stir in the garlic and simmer for around 1 minute, until fragrant. Sprinkle with salt and substitute the cherry tomatoes. Cook until the tomatoes start to burst, then add the spinach and cook until the spinach begins to wilt.

3. Stir in the heavy cream, basil and parmesan cheese and carry the mixture to a boil. Reduce the heat to low and boil for around 3 minutes before the sauce is significantly reduced.

4. Place the shrimp back in the pan and mix to blend. Cook unless shrimp is cooked through, garnish with more basil, and squeeze lemon on top before eating.

Zoodle Alfredo with Bacon

TOTAL TIME: 0 HOURS 20 MINS

YIELDS: 4

INGREDIENTS:

- 1/2 lb. of Chopped bacon
- 1 minced shallot,
- 2 garlic cloves, minced

- 1/4 c. of Black Alcohol, White Wine
- 1 1/2 c. of heavy cream
- 1/2 c. of Parmesan(cheese) grated, but mostly for garnishing
- 1 pack of zucchini (noodles) (16 oz.)
- Kosher Salt
- Black pepper freshly roast

DIRECTIONS

1. Cook the bacon until crisp, 8 minutes, in a wide saucepan over medium heat. Drain it on a tray lined with paper towels.

2. Pour all but 2 teaspoons of (bacon); then shallots are included. Cook until tender, around 2 minutes, and then add garlic and cook for about 30 seconds until it is fragrant. Add wine and cook before half the quantity is depleted.

3. Connect the heavy cream to the mixture and get it to a boil. Lower the flame and stir in the Parmesan cheese. Cook for about 2 minutes, until the sauce, has thick somewhat. Add the zucchini (noodles) and toss in the sauce until thoroughly covered. Take the heat off and stir in the fried bacon.

Keto Chicken Soup

TOTAL TIME: 1 HOUR 0 MINS

YIELDS: 4 - 6

INGREDIENTS:

- 2 tbsp. Oil for vegetables
- 1 medium onion, minced
- 5 garlic cloves, crushed
- 2" Fresh ginger bit, sliced
- 1 tiny cauliflower, sliced into florets
- 3/4 Tsp. smashed flakes of red pepper
- 1 medium carrot, on a bias, peeled and thin slices
- 6 c. low-sodium broth of poultry

- 1 celery stem, thinly sliced
- 2 skinless, boneless breasts of chicken
- For garnish, finely cut parsley

DIRECTIONS

1. Heat oil in a big pot over low heat. Add the carrot, ginger, and garlic. Cook before the browning stops.

2. In the meantime, pulse cauliflower before it is split into rice-sized granules in a food processor. Return the cauliflower to the pot with the onion mixture and cook for around 8 minutes over medium-high heat until golden.

3. Bring to a boil and incorporate pepper flakes, onions, celery and chicken (broth). Add the chicken breasts and cook gently for around 15 minutes before they hit a temp of 165 ° C. Remove from the pan, leave to cool and shred until cool enough to treat. Meanwhile, proceed to cook, 3 to 5 minutes more, until the vegetables are soft.

4. Apply the (Shredded) chicken back to the broth and cut the ginger from the bath. Season with salt and pepper to taste, then garnish before serving with parsley.

Foil Pack Grilled Salmon with Lemony Asparagus

TOTAL TIME: 0 HOURS **20** MINS

YIELDS: 4

INGREDIENTS:

- 20 spears of asparagus, cut

- 4 6-oz. Skin-on fillets of salmon

- 4Tbsp. of Butter, break

- 2 lemons, cut

- Kosher salt

- Black pepper freshly roasted

- Broken dill (fresh), for season

DIRECTIONS:

1. On a hard floor lie two bits of foil. Put on the foil five spears of asparagus and finish with a salmon fillet, 1 tablespoon of butter, and two lemon slices. Cover loosely, and repeat for the rest of the ingredients and you'll have a limit of four sets.

2. High Heat Barbecue. To fry and barbecue, apply foil packets until salmon is cook through and asparagus is soft for about 10 minutes.

3. Sprinkle and mix with dill.

Garlicky Shrimp Zucchini Pasta

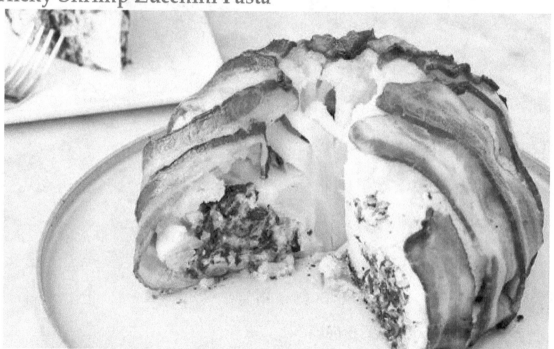

TOTAL TIME: 1 HOUR 50 MINS

YIELDS: 4

INGREDIENTS

- 1/4 c. Of olive oil extra-virgin
- 1/4 c. the Juice in Lemons

- Kosher (salt)
- 1 head (cauliflower), cut leaves and trimmed stem such that cauliflower lies flat but still intact
- 1 (10-oz.) box of frozen (spinach), thawed, stretched out and sliced with water
- 2 big, beaten eggs
- 4 green onions, cut thinly
  - 2 cloves of garlic, minced
  - 3/4 c. of cheddar Shredded
  - 4 oz. of soft and cube white cheese
  - 1/2 c. panko a panko
  - 1/4 c. of parmesan Rubbed
  - 1 lb. of bacon thinly cut

DIRECTIONS

1. Preheat the oven to 450 degrees. In a big kettle, put eight cups of water, oil, lemon juice and 2 tablespoons of salt to a boil. Add the cauliflower and get it to a simmer again. To hold it submerged, reduce it to a gentle simmer and put a plate on top of the cauliflower. Simmer for around 12 minutes before a knife is quickly inserted into the middle.

2. Transfer the cauliflower to a narrow rimmed baking sheet using 2 slotted spoons or a mesh spider. Only let it cool.

3. In the meanwhile, add lettuce (eggs, green onions, garlic, cheddar, cream cheese, panko, and parmesan cheese) and placed a 3/4-inch tip in a piping bag.

4. Place on a rimmed baking sheet with cooled cauliflower stem side up. Pipe filling of florets between stalks. Flip down the side of the cauliflower stem,

and then spread bacon strips, only slightly overlapping strips, over the cauliflower, tucking strip ends into the cauliflower bottom.

5. Roast, halfway through the spinning pan, before golden all over, maybe 30 minutes.

Cajun Parmesan Salmon

TOTAL TIME: 0 HOURS 45 MINS

YIELDS: 4

INGREDIENTS:

- 1 tbsp. Olive oil (extra-virgin)
- 4 (4-oz.) Salmon fillets (preferably wild)
- 2 Tsp. Seasoning the Cajun
- 2 Tbsp. of Butter

- 3 garlic cloves, minced
- 1/3 c. Low-sodium(chicken) or soup with vegetables
- Juice of 1 lemon
- 1 Tbsp. of honey
- 1 Tbsp. Freshly sliced parsley, with more for garnishing
- 2Tbsp. Parmesan, finely chopped
- Slices of lemon, for serving

DIRECTIONS

1. Heat oil in a frying pan over medium heat. Season the salmon with 1 tsp. of Cajun pepper and seasoning, then apply the skin-side-up to the skillet. Cook the salmon for around 6 minutes before it is intensely brown, then turn and cook for 2 more minutes. Transfer to a dish.

2. To the skillet, apply butter and garlic. Stir in the Broth, lemon juice, sugar, remaining Cajun seasoning teaspoon (parsley), and parmesan when the butter has melted. Take the combination to a boil.

3. Lower the heat to mild and return the salmon to the skillet. Simmer for 3 or 4 more minutes before the sauce is decreased, and the salmon is fried.

4. Apply slices of lemon to the pan and eat.

Beef Tenderloin:

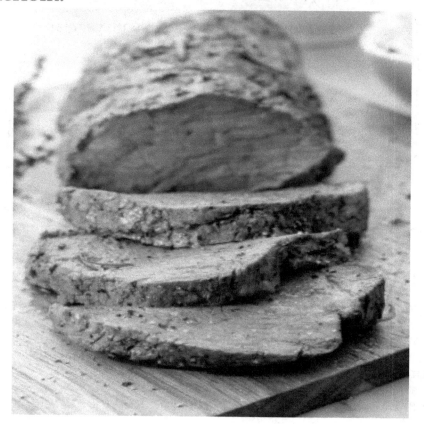

TOTAL TIME: 1 HOUR **50** MINS

YIELDS: 4

INGREDIENTS

FOR BEEF:

- 1/2 c. Olive oil (extra-virgin)
- 2 Tbsp. Vinegar (Balsamic)
- 2 Tbsp. Mustard, whole grain
- Thyme(fresh), 3 sprigs
- 3 rosemary sprigs, fresh
- 1 bay leaf

- 2 garlic cloves, crushed

- 2 tbsp. of honey

- 1 (2-lb.) tenderloin beef

- 1 Tsp. salt, Kosher

- 1 Tsp. Black pepper, roasted, fresh

- 1 Tsp. The Dried(Rosemary)

- 1 garlic clove, minced

- **SAUCE FOR YOGURT**

- 1/2 c. Yogurt (Greek)

- 1/4 c. Sour milk, sour cream

- 1 Tsp. Horseradish prepared

- 1/2 lemon extract

- Kosher salt

DIRECTIONS

1. Mix the vinegar, oil, thyme, mustard, rosemary, crushed garlic, bay leaf, and honey together in a wide container. Return the meat to the package, cover with plastic wrap, and marinate for 1 hour or up to one day in the refrigerator. Optional: Before frying, get the tenderloin to room temperature.

2. Preheat the oven to around 450C. Line an aluminum foil rimmed baking sheet and fit a wire rack inside. Strip the marinade from the tenderloin and wipe it dry with paper towels. Add salt, pepper, rosemary, and minced garlic to season all over and put on the rack.

3. Roast until baked to your taste, around 20 minutes for special occasions. Until slicing, let it rest for 5 to 10 minutes.

4. Meanwhile, render the sauce: whisk the milk, sour cream, horseradish and lemon juice together in a medium container, and season with salt.

5. Slice the tenderloin and eat it on the side with sauce.

Baked Cajun Salmon

TOTAL TIME: 0 HOURS 30 MINS

YIELDS: 4

INGREDIENTS

- 1/2 large size white onion, cut thinly

- bell pepper (red), cut thinly

- 1 thinly cut orange bell pepper

- cloves of thinly sliced garlic

- Salt (kosher)

- Black Pepper, fresh, ground

- Three Tbsp. of Olive Oil (Extra-Virgin)

- 1 Tbsp. of thyme in dry form

- 1 Tbsp. of seasoning (Cajun)

- 2 Tsp. Of tweet paprika

- Tsp. of powdered garlic

- 6-oz. Filets of Salmon

DIRECTIONS:

1. Preheat the oven to 400 degrees. Stir in the onions, pepper and garlic on a broad baking dish. Season with pepper and salt and toss with gasoline.

2. Prepare a spice mix: mix together thyme, Cajun seasoning, and paprika and garlic powder in a small cup.

3. On a baking sheet, put the salmon, top the bits with the seasoning mixture and rub them all over the salmon.

4. Bake for 20 minutes until the vegetables and salmon are soft and cooked properly.

Chapter 5: Deserts and Snacks Recipes

Keto Sugar-Free Cheesecake

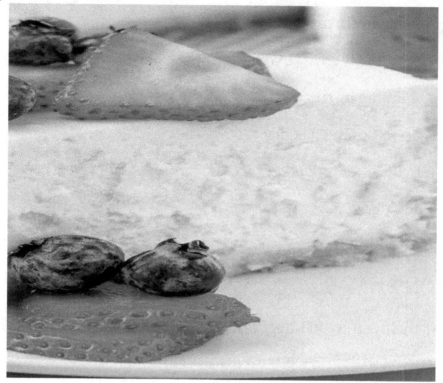

TOTAL TIME: 8 HOURS 0 MINS

YIELDS: 8 - 10

INGREDIENTS:

- 1/2 c. of almond flour
- 1/2 c. Flour of coconut
- 1/4 c. of coconut, shredded
- 1/2 c. (1 stick) of melted butter
- 3 (8-oz.) cream cheese blocks, soft to room temp
- 16 oz. of sour cream (room temperature)
- 1 Tbsp. of stevia

- 2 Tsp. a sample of pure vanilla
- 3 large size eggs, at room temperature
- Strawberries, diced, for serving

DIRECTIONS

1. Heat the oven to 300 degrees. Create the crust: Oil a spring pan of 8 or 9 inches and coat the bottom and sides with foil. Mix the rice, coconut, and butter together in a medium dish. Push the crust towards the bottom and the sides of the prepared pan somewhat upwards. When you prepare the filling, put the pan in the fridge.

2. Prepare the filling: mix together the cream cheese and sour cream in a large bowl, then whisk in the stevia and vanilla. One at a time, add the eggs, combining after each addition. Layer the filling over the crust uniformly.

3. Put the cheesecake in a deep roasting pan and set it on the oven's center rack. Pour sufficient boiling water carefully into the roasting pan to come halfway up the spring type pan's sides. Bake for 1 hour to 1 hour 20 minutes, until the middle jiggles just slightly. Switch off the oven, but allow the cake to cool steadily for an hour in the oven with the door partially closed.

4. Remove the pan from the boiling water, remove the foil, and then let it cool for at least five hours or overnight in the refrigerator. Slice with the strawberries and garnish.

Keto Chocolate Chip Cookies

TOTAL TIME: 0 HOURS 30 MINS

YIELDS: 18

INGREDIENTS:

- 2 large size eggs

- 1/2 c (1 stick) of butter that has melted

- 2 Tbsp. of heavy milk to heavy cream

- 2 Tsp .pure extract of vanilla

- 2 3/4 c. of almond flour

- 1/4 Tsp. salt, kosher

- 1/4 c. Sugar granulated keto-friendly (such as swerve)

- 3/4 c. Chips of dark chocolate (such as lily's)

- cooking mist

DIRECTIONS

1. Preheat 350° in the oven. Mix the egg with the sugar, vanilla and heavy cream in a big dish. Add the almond flour, salt and swerve to the mixture.

2. Fold in the cookie batter with the chocolate chips. Shape the mixture into 1" balls and arrange 3" apart on baking sheets lined with parchment. Flatten the balls with cooking spray on the bottom of a glass that has been oiled.

3. Bake for around 17 to 19 minutes until the cookies are softly golden.

Keto Chocolate Mug Cake

TOTAL TIME: 0 HOURS 5 MINS

YIELDS: 1

INGREDIENTS:

- 2 Tbsp. of Butter
- 1/4 c. of almond flour
- 2 Tbsp. of powdered cocoa
- 1 large size egg, beaten
- 2 Tbsp. of chocolate chips that are keto-friendly, (such as Lily's)
- 2 Tbsp. of Swerve, Granulated
- 1/2 Tsp. of baking powder
- A pinch of Kosher salt
- For serving, whipped cream (1/4 c.)

DIRECTIONS

1. Put the butter in a microwave-safe mug and heat for 30 seconds before it is melted. Except for whipped cream, add the remaining ingredients and stir until thoroughly mixed. Cook until the cake is set, but always fudgy, for 45 seconds to 1 minute.

2. Serve with whipped cream.

Keto Ice Cream

TOTAL TIME: 8 HOURS 15 MINS

YIELDS: 8

INGREDIENT:

- 2 cans of coconut milk (15-oz.)
- 2 c. of heavy cream
- 1/4 c. Swerve the Sweetener of the Confectioner
- 1 Tsp. of pure vanilla
- A pinch of Kosher salt

DIRECTIONS

1. In the refrigerator, chill the coconut milk for at least 3 hours, preferably overnight.

2. To make whipped coconut: pour coconut cream into a big bowl, keep liquid in the bowl and beat the coconut cream until very smooth using a hand mixer. Only put back.

3. Make the whipped cream: Using a hand mixer in a separate big bowl (or a stand mixer in a bowl), beat heavy cream until soft peaks shape. Beat in the vanilla and sweetener.

4. Fold the whipped (coconut) into the whipped cream, and then add the mixture to the loaf plate.

5. Freeze for about 5 hours until it is firm.

Keto Hot Chocolate

TOTAL TIME: 0 HOURS 10 MINS

YIELDS: 1 CUP

INGREDIENTS:

- 2 Tbsp. Powder of unsweetened chocolate, and more for garnishing
- 2 1/2 Tsp. of sugar that is keto-friendly, such as Swerve
- 1 1/4 c. Aquatic Water
- 1/4 c. Heavy milk to heavy cream
- 1/4 Tsp. of pure vanilla
- Whipped(milk),for serving

DIRECTIONS:

1. Whisk together the swerve, chocolate, and about 2 teaspoons of water in a shallow pan over medium heat until smoother and dissolve. Increases heat to low, add the remaining cream and water and whisk until heated regularly.
2. Attach the vanilla, and spill it into a cup. Represent with (whipped) cream and chocolate powder dusting.

Keto Peanut Butter Cookies

TOTAL TIME: 1 HOUR 30 MINS

YIELDS: 22

INGREDIENTS

- 1 1/2c. of smooth peanut butter, unsweetened, melted (plus more for drizzling)

- 1 c. Flour of coconut

- 1/4 c. Keto-friendly brown sugar packets, such as Swerve

- 1 Tsp. of pure vanilla

- Pinch of Kosher salt

- 2 c. of melted keto-friendly dark chocolate chips, including Lily's,

- 1 Tbsp. of Cream (Coconut)

-

DIRECTIONS

1. Combine the sugar, coconut flour, peanut butter, salt, and vanilla in a medium dish. Until smooth, stir.

2. Line the parchment paper with a baking sheet. Shape the mixture into circles using a small cookie scoop, then push down gently to flatten slightly and position it on the baking sheet. Freeze until strong, roughly 1 hour.

3. Whisk the melting chocolate and coconut oil together in a medium dish.

4. Dip peanut butter rounds in chocolate using a fork until fully covered and then return to the baking sheet. Drizzle with much more peanut butter, and freeze for around 10 minutes before the chocolate is set.

5. Only serve it cold. In the fridge, put some leftovers.

Chocolate Keto Cookies

TOTAL TIME: 0 HOURS 25 MINS

YIELDS: 11

INGREDIENTS

- 2 1/2 Tbsp. of butter

- 3 Tbsp. of chocolate chips with keto, split

- 1large size egg

- 1 Tsp. of pure vanilla

- 2/3 of c. Almond Flour Blanched

- 1/3 c. of swerve Confectioners

- 3 1/2 Tbsp. Unsweetened dark chocolate powder

- 1/2 Tsp. Powder used for baking

- Pinch of Kosher salt

DIRECTIONS

1. Preheat the oven to 325 degrees. Add butter and half of the (chocolate chips) into a medium-sized dish. Microwave for 15 to 30 seconds, only enough time to melt the chocolate and butter mildly. Until a chocolate sauce emerges, mix the two together.

2. Attach and whisk the egg in a tiny dish before the yolk mixes with the whites. When it's finished, add the chocolate syrup to the bowl with the egg and vanilla extract. Again, blend.

3. To finish the cookies, add the majority of the dry ingredients, save some of the chocolate chips. Mix until it shapes a mass of chocolate cookie dough.

4. To make 11 equal-sized cookies, use a cookie spoon (or a tablespoon). Attach the cookie to a baking parchment paper and top the remainder of the chocolate chips with each cookie. In either a spoon or a spatula, flatten each cookie.

5. For 8 to 10 minutes, roast. When they come out of the oven, they should be very soft, but don't worry, this is natural!

6. Let the cookies on the baking sheet cool off. They can set up and firm up while they cool up.

7. When the leftovers are cooled, enjoy them and store them in an airtight jar in the refrigerator.

Walnut Snowball Cookies:

TOTAL TIME: 1 HOUR 5 MINS

YIELDS: 15

INGREDIENTS

- 1/2 c. (1 stick) of butter that has melted

- 1 large size egg

- 50 drops of stevia liquid (about 1/4 tsp.)

- 1/2 tsp. of pure vanilla

- 1 c. With walnuts

- 1/2 c. Flour of coconut, plus 1 or 2 tbsp. For rolling, more

- 1/2 c. of swerve Confectioners

DIRECTIONS

1. Preheat the oven to 300 ° and use parchment paper to cover a baking sheet. In a large bowl, mix the melted butter, egg, vanilla extract, stevia and set aside.

2. In a food processor, add the walnuts and pulse until ground. In a medium bowl, pour the walnut flour and add the coconut flour and 1/4 cup Swerve and press until mixed.

3. Add the dry mixture to the wet in two sections and whisk to blend. The dough should be soft but strong enough at this stage to shape hand-made balls without sticking to your hands. If the quality is not right, add 1 to 2 tablespoons of extra (coconut) flour and mix.

4. Create 15 balls of the same size and place them on a lined baking sheet. In the microwave, they would not disperse.

5. For 30 minutes, roast.

6. Enable 5 minutes to settle, and then in the remaining 1/4 cup Swerve, roll the (still warm) spheres.

7. Put them back on the parchment paper and give another 20 to 30 minutes to cool fully before feeding.

Keto Tortilla Chips

TOTAL TIME: 0 HOURS 35 MINS

YIELDS: 4 - 6

INGREDIENTS

- 2 c. of Mozzarella cheese, Sliced
- 1 c. of almond flour
- 1 Tsp. salt, Kosher
- 1 Tsp. of garlic powder
- 1/2 Tsp. Powdered chili
- Black pepper freshly ground

DIRECTIONS

1. Preheat the oven to 350 degrees. Top the parchment paper with two wide baking sheets.

2. Melt the mozzarella in a secure microwave bowl for around 1 minute and 30 seconds. Add the almond flour, cinnamon, chili powder, garlic powder, black pepper and a few pieces. Use both hands to moisten the dough a couple of times before it forms a smooth shape.

3. Place the dough between two parchment paper sheets and stretch it out into a 1/8' wide rectangle. Break the dough into triangles using a knife or a pizza cutter.

4. Spread the chips on lined baking sheets and bake for 12 to 14 minutes until the sides are golden and begin to crisp.

Keto Burger Fat Bombs

TOTAL TIME: 0 HOURS 30 MINS

YIELDS: 20

INGREDIENTS:

- Cooking mist
- 1 lb. of meat, ground
- 1/2 tsp. powder in garlic form
- salt (kosher)
- Black pepper freshly ground
- 2 tbsp. Cold butter, 20 bits of sliced butter
- 2 oz. Split into 20 bits of cheddar,
- Lettuce berries meant for serving
- For serving, finely sliced tomatoes
- Mustard, to serve

DIRECTIONS

1. Preheat the oven to 375 °C and oil the cooking spray with a mini muffin tin. Season the beef with salt, garlic powder and pepper in a medium dish.

2. Place 1 teaspoon of beef equally, covering the bottom entirely, into the bottom of each muffin tin cup. Place a slice of butter on top and press 1 teaspoon of beef over the butter to cover full.

3. In each cup, place a slice of cheddar on top of the meat and force the remaining beef over the cheese to cover it fully.

4. Bake for about 15 minutes before the meat is ready. Let yourself cool somewhat.

5. Using a metal offset spatula carefully to release each burger out of the tin. Serve with onions, salad leaves, and mustard.

Jalapeño Popper Egg Cups

TOTAL TIME: 0 HOURS 45 MINS

YIELDS: 12

INGREDIENTS:

- 12 strips of bacon
- 10 eggs (large)
- 1/4 c. of sour milk,
- 1/2 c. Cheddar Shredded
- 1/2 c. Mozzarella Sliced
- 2(jalapeños), 1 sliced thinly and 1 finely chopped
- 1 Tsp. Powdered of garlic
- salt(kosher)
- Black pepper freshly ground

- Cooking spray, nonstick

DIRECTIONS

1. Preheat the oven to 375 degrees. Over medium heat, (cook bacon) in a broad skillet until well browned but always pliable. Put aside to drain on a paper towel-lined pan.

2. Whisk the eggs, sour cream, cheese, minced jalapeño and garlic in powder form together in a big bowl. With salt and pepper, season.

3. Oil a muffin tin with the aid of nonstick cooking oil. Line each well with one bacon strip, then pour each muffin cup with egg mixture until around two-thirds of the way through to the end. Cover each muffin with a slice of jalapeño.

4. Bake for 20 minutes until the eggs do not look moist anymore. Before withdrawing them from the muffin pan, cool slightly.

Keto Frosty

TOTAL TIME: 0 HOURS 45 MINS

YIELDS: 4

INGREDIENTS

- 1 1/2 c. Heavy cream whipping
- 2 Tbsp. Unsweetened powder of cocoa
- 3 Tbsp. Sweetener for (keto-friendly) powdered sugar, such as a Swerve
- 1 Tsp. of pure vanilla
- Pinch of Kosher salt

DIRECTIONS

1. Combine the milk, sugar, sweetener, vanilla, and salt in a wide pot. Beat the mixture until rigid peaks shape, and use a hand blender or (the whisk attachment of a stand mixer). Mix the scoops into a Ziploc container and ice for 30 to 35 minutes before they're frozen.
2. Break the tip off an edge of the Ziploc container and pour it into dishes to eat.

Bacon Guac Bombs

TOTAL TIME: 0 HOURS 45 MINS

YIELDS: 15

INGREDIENTS:

2 bacon strips, fried and crumbled

For guacamole

- 2 pitted, sliced, and mashed avocados
- 6 oz. of Cream cheese, cooked, softened
- 1 lime juice
- 1 clove of garlic, minced
- 1/4 of red onion, minced
- 1 small jalapeno (seeded if less fire is preferred), chopped
- 2 Tbsp. Cilantro, freshly sliced

- 1/2 Tsp. of cumin seeds
- 1/2 Tsp. Powdered of chili
- salt(kosher)
- Black pepper freshly ground

DIRECTIONS

1. Combine all the guacamole products in a big bowl. Stir unless mostly smooth, and add salt and pepper (some pieces are OK). Put in the freezer for 30 minutes to firm up rapidly.

2. On a wide tray, put crumbled bacon. Scoop the guacamole mix and put in the bacon, utilizing a little cookie scoop. Roll in the bacon to coat. Repeat before you've used both the bacon and guacamole. Store in refrigerator.

Avocado Chips

TOTAL TIME: 0 HOURS 40 MINS

YIELDS: 15

INGREDIENTS

- 1 large ripe avocado
- 3/4 c. Freshly grated parmesan
- 1 tsp. Lemon juice
- 1/2 tsp. Garlic powder
- 1/2 tsp. Italian seasoning
- Kosher salt
- Freshly ground black pepper

DIRECTIONS

1. Preheat oven to 325° and line two baking sheets with parchment paper. In a medium bowl, mash avocado with a fork until smooth. Stir in parmesan, lemon juice, garlic powder, and Italian seasoning. Season with salt and pepper.

2. Place heaping teaspoon-size scoops of mixture on baking sheet, leaving about 3" apart between each scoop. Flatten each scoop to 3" wide across with the back of a spoon or measuring cup. Bake until crisp and golden, about 30 minutes, then let cool completely. Serve at room temperature.

Rosemary Keto Crackers

TOTAL TIME: 1 HOUR 0 MINS

YIELDS: 140

INGREDIENTS

- 2 1/2 c. almond flour

- 1/2 c. coconut flour
- 1 tsp. ground flaxseed meal
- 1/2 tsp. dried rosemary, chopped
- 1/2 tsp. onion powder
- 1/4 tsp. kosher salt
- 3 large eggs
- 1 tbsp. extra-virgin olive oil

DIRECTIONS

1. Preheat oven to 325° and line a baking sheet with parchment paper. In a large bowl, whisk together flours, flaxmeal, rosemary, onion powder, and salt. Add eggs and oil and mix to combine. Continue mixing until dough forms a large ball, about 1 minute.

2. Sandwich dough between 2 pieces of parchment and roll to ¼" thick. Cut into squares and transfer to prepared baking sheet.

3. Bake until golden, 12 to 15 minutes. Let cool before storing in a resalable container.

Conclusion

A ketogenic diet could be an alternative for certain people who have experienced trouble losing weight with other approaches. The exact ratio of fat, carbohydrate, and protein that is required to attain health benefits can differ among individuals due to their genetic makeup and body structure. Therefore, if one decides to start a ketogenic diet, it is advised to meet with one's physician and a dietitian to closely track any metabolic adjustments since beginning the treatment and to develop a meal schedule that is specific to one's current health problems and to avoid food shortages or other health risks. A dietitian can also have advice on reintroducing carbs after weight reduction is accomplished.

Intermittent Fasting for Women

Look Better, Fell Better and Discover a Modern Approach to Autophagy to Thrive in a Post Pandemic Scenario

By

Casey Black

Table of Contents

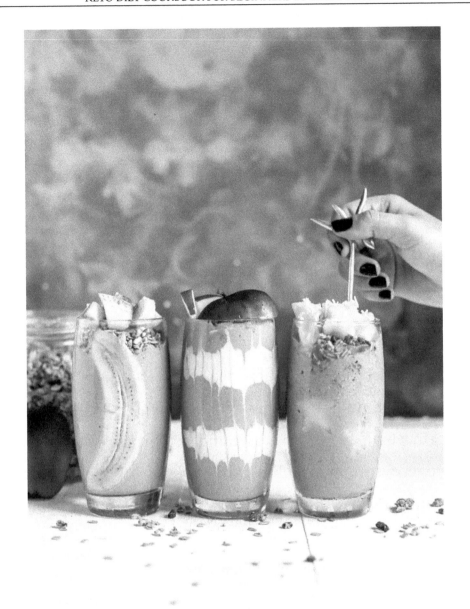

Introduction

Congratulations on downloading Intermittent Fasting for women: *The Ultimate Beginners Guide for Permanent Weight Loss, Slow the Aging Process, and Heal Your Body with the Self-cleansing Process of Metabolic Autophagy.*

This book is your ultimate guide to intermittent fasting. In this book, you'll explore everything about intermittent fasting; what it is, how it works, and how best you can adapt it to suit your needs as a woman. The intermittent fasting diet is one of the best ways to lose weight since it's not restrictive but instead advocates for a change in lifestyle.

You'll notice that this book covers many facets of intermittent fasting, thus offering as much guidance you need to help you get started. This book also discredits the common belief that breakfast is the most important meal of the days hence can't be skipped. Moreover, nutritionists will tell you to eat multiple small meals during the day to stay healthy, but the intermittent fasting diet overrides this principle. The science behind the intermittent fasting is backed by various research studies that have proved that you can actually skip breakfast.

We all have a tendency to naturally fast that makes it easy to integrate intermittent fasting into our lifestyles. In fact, once you adjust to your new lifestyle of intermittent fasting, you'll be surprised that you actually don't eat as much as you think you do or you need to. Intermittent fasting will help you to not only fulfill your weight loss goals but also meet your dietary needs, fight off diseases, and maintain a healthy lifestyle.

Even then, as you read this book keep in mind that everyone's experience with intermittent fasting is different. This is the key to implementing it in your life because you'll find it easy to stick to the intermittent fasting plan that is convenient for you. It's never too late to make significant changes to your lifestyle with intermittent fasting. You can begin today.

Chapter 1: Obesity and Its Impact on Women

Obesity has a negative impact on the health of women, yet 2 in 3 women in the United States are obese. What is obesity, and how do you know you are obese? Obesity is a disorder that is characterized by having an excessive amount of body fat. It is diagnosed when your body mass index is (BMI) 30 or higher. This is calculated by dividing your weight in kilograms by your height in meters squared. Wondering what your BMI is? Can you use online BMI calculators to find out your BMI? Even then, BMI is considered less accurate in some people, especially if you're very muscular since muscles weigh more than fat. The other ways to find out if your weight is healthy is by measuring your waist circumference. If your waist circumference is more than 35 inches, then you have a higher risk of experiencing the problems associated with obesity.

Your body needs calories to work properly. However, when your body is storing more calories than its burning over time, you become obese because it means you're gaining weight. However, environmental factors can also influence obesity. When you are extremely obese, you are likely to have a myriad of health problems in addition to having low self-esteem. As a woman, you are also at risk of suffering from diseases like diabetes, heart disease, and even certain types of cancers.

Obesity Risk Factors

Although women of all ages, ethnicities, and races can be obese, obesity tends to be more common among African American Women and Latina or Hispanic women. Other risk factors for obesity among women include the following:

Genetics and family background. For some people, obesity runs in the family. This is not to say that there's a single fat gene. Rather, many genes work together resulting in your likelihood of gaining excess weight. Additionally, the kind of food you're given as a child by your caregivers and parents can influence your weight gain as an adult.

Metabolism. The rate at which your body breaks down calories will often vary from one person to the other due to various reasons affecting your weight loss and gain. When you have more muscle and less fat, your body burns fat quickly. On the contrary, when you have more fat and less muscle, you're more likely to gain weight. Moreover, your metabolism may also be affected by hormonal changes at puberty, during pregnancy, and when you get into menopause.

Trauma. You may sometimes go through life issues that you don't have control over or are not your fault that affects how fast you gain weight. Women who experience negative events in their childhood like alcoholic parents or abuse are more likely to be obese as adults.

Sleep: Lack of high-quality sleep could also lead to weight gain. This is because not getting quality sleep can affect your hormone levels, which eventually has an effect on your food choices and appetite. Not getting enough sleep may also affect your level or exercise and physical activity throughout the day.

Medicines. Some of the medicines that you may be taking such as those used in treating mental health conditions, high blood pressure, and sleep can lead to weight gain. Medicines may also make it difficult to lose weight. If you're taking prescription medicine and you notice you're gaining extra weight, don't hesitate to talk to your doctor to give you alternative medicine or ways of losing weight.

With so many factors contributing to unhealthy weight gain, you always have to be alert to know what is making you gain weight to make sure you keep your weight under control. When you're overweight or obese, it increases your risk of having serious health conditions such as:

Cancer. Women who are obese have a high risk of suffering from various types of cancer such as cancer of the thyroid, ovarian, pancreatic, multiple myeloma (blood plasma cells), meningioma (cancer of tissue covering spinal cord and brain, kidney, liver, stomach, esophagus, endometrial, colon, rectal, breast and gall bladder.

Breathing problems. When you're overweight, you'll most likely experience sleep apnea. This causes you to stop breathing or take in slow breaths during sleep. Consequently, you'll not get enough oxygen in your body or brain during sleep. This can lead to more serious health issues like heart disease.

Heart disease. Your risk of having heart disease increases with excess weight. Therefore, you must strive to keep your weight in check in order to stay healthy and avoid heart disease that is a leading cause of death among women.

Diabetes. Having extra weight predisposes you to diabetes. On the contrary, you can prevent diabetes when you lose weight or keep your weight within the recommended range. Weight loss is also important in controlling your blood glucose, especially if you already suffer from diabetes. In fact, you'll less likely need medicine to keep your blood sugar in control.

Pregnancy problems. You might find it difficult getting pregnant when you are obese. If you're already pregnant, you're likely to experience complications like preeclampsia (dangerously high blood pressure) and gestational diabetes. Thus, you'll need close monitoring and regular prenatal care to ensure early detection and prevention of such problems.

High blood pressure. If you've obesity, you're more likely to have high blood pressure and may be advised by your doctor to lose some weight to reduce your blood pressure. When you have high blood pressure, it can damage your arteries resulting in related health conditions like heart disease and stroke.

Stroke. Being obese increases your chances of suffering from a stroke. This is particularly serious when most of your weight is around your waist than thighs and hips.

High cholesterol. When your weight is more excess, your body will change the way it processes food. Thus, your bad cholesterol increases while your good cholesterol is reduced. Consequently, the buildup of fatty plaque increases within your arteries. An increase in bad cholesterol can lead to heart disease.

You need to know when to start working towards losing weight. A 3 to 5 % loss is capable of helping lower your risk of health problems while making you healthier. Therefore, take time to discuss with your doctor the amount of weight you must lose.

Chapter 2: The Skinny on Intermittent Fasting

Losing excessive body weight/fat can be a challenge. In most cases, you'll have to give up something you love and embrace a change of lifestyle by hitting the gym. But did you know that you can lose fat, improve your metabolism, and enjoy all the other health benefits without giving up the foods you love? Intermittent fasting is an incredible solution to shedding off excess fat that comes with other benefits you'll enjoy. So, what is intermittent fasting? Although most people think of it as a diet, it is not. Intermittent fasting is a pattern of eating that cycles between periods of eating and fasting and has been proven to be effective in weight loss while sustaining the results.

Interestingly, intermittent fasting is a practice that has been in existence for a long time. What makes intermittent fasting unique is the way in which you schedule your meals. You don't change what you eat, instead what changes are when you eat. That is, instead of dictating the foods you should eat, it dictates when you should eat. Thus, with intermittent fasting, you get lean and building your muscle mass without cutting down your calories. Even then, most people opt for intermittent fasting for the sole reason of losing fat.

Who Invented the Intermittent Fasting Diet

Fasting is not a new thing. It has been practiced since human evolution. In fact, the human body is wired to fast. The hunter and gatherer population did have much food to store, and they would sometimes have nothing to eat due to scarcity. As such, they adopted the ability to function without food for long periods that are essentially fasting. There's also a religious angle to fasting for Christians and Muslims alike.

However, the current wave of intermitted fasting diet was popularized by Dr. Michael Mosley. Intermittent fasting has generated a steady positive buzz with more and more people embracing it. Dr. Mosley explains the science behind intermittent fasting. He, however, attributes the success and popularity of intermittent fasting to the fact that it's mostly psychological and teaches you better ways of eating. That is, when you get used to eating vegetables and good protein, you'll eventually crave healthy food whenever you're hungry.

Why Do You Fast

Intermittent fasting is a simple yet effective strategy for taking shedding off all the bad weight so that you only keep the good weight. This approach requires very little change in behavior. Thus, it's simple yet meaningful enough to make a difference. When you fast, a couple of changes take place in your body both at the molecular and cellular level. To understand why you need to fast to lose weight, you first must understand what happens to your body when it is in the fed and absorptive state. In the fed state, your body is absorbing and digesting food. It actually begins when you start eating and would typically last for five hours as digestion and absorption of the food you ate takes place. When your body is in this state, it can hardly burn fat due to high insulin levels. From the fed state, your body enters the postabsorptive state during which no meal processing is taking place. This stage lasts between 8 and 12 hours after the last meal before you enter the fasted state. It is during the fasted state that your body burns fat because your insulin levels are low. In the fasted state, your body burns fat that is usually inaccessible in the fed state. Fasting helps to put your body in the fat burning state that is rare to achieve when you're on a normal eating schedule.

Intermittent fasting changes the hormones in your body to utilize your fat stores effectively. Your human growth hormone levels go up dramatically, thus speeding up protein synthesis, thereby influencing your body's fat loss and muscle gain by making the fat available for use as a source of energy. What this means is that your body will be burning fat and packing muscle faster. When your insulin levels drop due to heightened insulin sensitivity making the fat stored in your body more accessible to be converted to energy, some changes in gene functions relating to protection and longevity will be amplified, and your cells will initiate repair processes efficiently and quickly. Moreover, fasting promotes autophagy that removes all the damaged cells while contributing to the renewal of cells in addition to supporting the body's regenerative processes.

What You Should Eat During Intermittent Fasting

One of the reasons why intermittent fasting is appealing is because there are no food rules. The only restrictions are on when you can eat and not what you can eat. However, this is not to say that you should be downing bags of chips and pints upon pints of ice cream. Remember, the idea is to adopt a healthy eating lifestyle. So what should you eat anyway? Well, a well-balanced diet is key to maintaining your energy levels. If your goal is to lose weight, you must focus on including nutrient-dense foods on your menu like veggies, fruits, nuts, whole grains, seeds, beans, lean proteins, and dairy. Think about unprocessed, high fiber, whole foods that offer flavor and variety. Here are some foods you should eat in plenty during intermittent fasting:

Water. Although you're not eating, it's important to make sure your stay hydrated to maintain the health of major organs in the body. To tell if you have adequate water, make sure your urine is pale yellow. Dark urine is a sign of dehydration that can cause fatigue, headaches, or even lightheadedness. If you can't stand plain water, you can add mint leaves, a squeeze of lemon juice or cucumber slices.

Fish. Dietary guidelines advocate for the consumption of at least eight ounces of fish weekly. Fish is a rich source of protein, ample quantities of Vitamin D and healthy fats. Moreover, limiting your calorie consumption can alter your cognitive ability; hence, fish will come in handy as brain food.

Avocado. It's obviously strange to eat high-calorie food when you're actually trying to lose weight. Well, the thing about avocadoes is that they're packed with monounsaturated fat that is satiating. Thus, you can be sure to stay full for longer hours than you would when you eat other foods.

Cruciferous vegetables. Foods like Brussels sprouts, broccoli, and cauliflower, are laden with fiber. Eating these foods will keep you regular while preventing constipation. Furthermore, you'll also fee full, which is great when you're fasting for hours.

Beans and legumes. Carbs are a great source of energy; hence, you can consider including low-calorie carbs like legumes and beans in your eating plan. Besides, foods like black beans, lentils, and chickpeas have been found to decrease body weight.

Potatoes. Potatoes are not necessarily bad. If anything, they offer a satiating effect that could lead to weight loss. However, this doesn't include potato chips and French fries.

Eggs. It's important to get as much protein as possible to build muscle and stay full. A large egg will give you six grams of proteins. When you eat hard boiled eggs, you're less likely to feel hungry.

Berries. You need immune boosting nutrients like vitamin c, and there's no better way to achieve this than including berries in your meal plan.

Probiotics. The bacteria in your gut aren't happy when you go for hours without food. As such, you could experience side effects like constipation. You can counter this unpleasant feeling taking probiotic-rich foods like kefir, kraut, or kombucha.

Whole grains. It's ridiculous to be on a diet and eat carbs. Well, with intermittent fasting, you can include whole grains that are rich in protein and fiber to stay full. Moreover, eating whole grains will speed up your metabolism. Think about millet, amaranth, sorghum, kamut, spelled, faro, bulgur, and freekeh, among others.

Nuts. Although nuts may contain high calories, they're most certainly important because of the good fat. According to research, polyunsaturated fat found in walnuts has the ability to alter physiological markers for satiety and hunger.

What to Consider Before Starting Intermittent Fasting

Before you begin intermittent fasting for weight loss, you need to know that this eating pattern is not for everyone. First off, you should not attempt intermittent fasting before consulting a health professional if you're underweight or you have a history of battling eating disorders. Intermittent fasting is also not recommended if you have a medical condition. Some women have also reported various effects like a cessation of a menstrual period. Ultimately, you need to be careful when you go into intermittent fasting because it has been previously found that this eating pattern is not beneficial for women compared to men. If you have fertility issues or are trying to conceive, then consider holding off intermittent fasting. Expectant and lactating mothers are also advised against intermittent fasting.

The main side effect that you'll experience when you go into intermittent fasting is hunger. Additionally, you may experience general body weakness. Your brain may also perform well. However, these are temporary, and your body will adapt to your new eating pattern over time. It's advisable that you consult your doctor before starting intermittent fasting for women if you have any of the following conditions;

• Diabetes/Problems with blood sugar regulations

• Low blood pressure

• You are underweight

• Eating disorders

• Amenorrhea

• Breastfeeding

• Trying to conceive

• Taking medications

Always look at the potential benefits of intermittent fasting before you go for it. If the risks far outweigh the benefits, this could be dangerous hence not worth trying. For instance, if you're pregnant, you definitely have more energy needs; therefore, taking on intermittent fasting would definitely be a bad idea. This also applies when you're having problems sleeping or are under chronic stress. Intermittent fasting is also discouraged if you have a history of eating disorders because it could actually cause further problems that can mess your health. While intermittent fasting has produced results for thousands of people across the globe, you must keep in mind that this is not a gateway to eating a diet comprising of highly processed food or even skipping meals randomly. Generally, intermittent fasting has an outstanding safety profile since it's not dangerous to go without food for a while when you're well-nourished and healthy.

When Do You Fast

If you're looking to get on the intermittent fasting train, you need to know when you will be fasting in order to achieve the desired outcome. There are three common ways of approaching the fast as follows:

Eat stop eat. This involves fasting for 24 hours once or twice in seven days. However, you can take calorie-free beverages during this fasting period. This is one of the best ways to start intermittent fasting because the occasional fasting will equally help you realize the many benefits of fasting.

Up day, down day. With this method of fasting, you will keep on reducing your calorie intake daily. That is, when you eat very little one day (down day), you revert to your normal caloric intake the next day (up day). The advantage of this eating pattern is that it allows you to eat every day while you still reap the benefits of fasting.

Alternate day fasting. With this schedule, you get to fast for longer periods on alternate days weekly. You fast for 24 hours and only eat one meal every day.

Lean gains. With this approach, you'll fast for 16 hours within every 24 hours and only eat during the eight-hour window. Keep in mind that sleep is included so this is not as tough as it may seem. The good thing about this fast is that you can start your 8-hour eating period at a time that works best for you. This means that you could actually skip breakfast and instead have lunch and dinner. Since this is something you'll do every day, it eventually becomes a habit making it remarkably easy to stick to it.

Chapter 3: Why Intermittent Fasting Is the Best Way for Weight Loss

Most of the weight loss diet fads will often demand that you give up certain things in order for you to see the results. Well, this is not the case with intermittent fasting that almost blends into your normal eating and sleeping pattern. Even then, the truth is that fasting in itself can be intimidating. Not eating for a couple of hours is something many people find difficult. Yet this method comes close to your lifestyle than a diet. So make sure that you identify an intermittent fasting plan that fits into your schedule, and you're able to keep up with comfortably. This will minimize the chance of having to quit because you're not putting any strain on your body.

Think about this; you fast while sleeping and break the fast when you wake up in the morning! Even more interesting, most people often fast for 12 hours and have another 12 hours of eating. As such, you can easily extend the fasting window to 16 hours and eat for eight hours to realize the benefits of intermittent fasting. Here are reasons why you should consider intermittent fasting as your weight loss regime:

Intermittent fasting is convenient. One of the reasons many people give up on other kinds of weight loss diets is because they're unable to follow through. When you have a busy lifestyle juggling between a number of things that are vying for your attention and are on a diet, the latter will definitely suffer.

On the contrary, intermittent fasting comes with convenience. For instance, when doing the 16:8 intermittent fast, you don't have to think about preparing breakfast in the morning or even lunch. Yes, you can skip breakfast.

What's more? When it's time to feed, you don't have to worry about what kind of food you should eat. Intermittent fasting is quite flexible with the foods you can include in your diet. In fact, in most instances, nothing will really change. You could even eat at a restaurant yet still enjoy the benefits of fasting.

Moreover, intermittent fasting lets you enjoy special occasions with family and friends without worrying about excess calories. However, this does not mean that you eat highly processed foods. The idea here is to develop a healthy yet convenient to implement eating pattern that can eventually be part of your lifestyle.

Intermittent fasting makes life simple. Intermittent fasting is not just convenient but also simple to follow. Whether you're always on the go or are into skipping a meal or two, this eating pattern is convenient and perfect for you. College students will particularly find intermittent fasting appealing because they can hardly find a balance between school work and maintaining a healthy social life. When you take on intermittent fasting, you'll realize there'll be fewer decisions you have to make daily. Instead, you'll have more energy to handle the most important tasks of the day. This is contrary to the effect that most diets will have on your body like feeling overwhelmed and tired in addition to being expensive and complex.

Intermittent fasting saves you time and money. If you were to go on a regular diet, no doubt you'll have to go out of your way to spend time and money to conform to a certain menu. Not to mention the amount of time that would go into shopping for the food supplies, prepping and eventually cooking at least six meals in a day. The truth is that this can be draining. However, with intermittent fasting, there's no need to get out of your normal lifestyle. If anything, it will save you money and time since you'll be having fewer meals in a day. Consequently, you don't have to spend time thinking about what you should eat or even spending a lot of time preparing the food.

Intermittent fasting strengthens your will power while improving your concentration and focus. Intermittent fasting is all about self-discipline. That is, you must learn to say no. In fact, there'll be numerous times during your fast when you'll crave food, but you must resist this urge to eat. Every time you resist this urge helps you develop your willpower as well as strengthen your ability to steer clear of distractions and temptations even in other areas of life. In addition, it'll also go a long way in improving your ability to focus and concentrate on achieving specific goals that you have yet to accomplish. Generally, you tend to be sharper and alert when you're hungry than when you've got a full tummy. This is attributed to the fact that fasting will free up all the valuable energy hence avoiding distractions while staying focused on an important goal.

Intermittent fasting lets you eat what you want and still lose weight. With intermittent fasting, weight loss is more about when you eat as opposed to what you eat. As such, it gives you more freedom to eat what you want to eat. Since you're fasting, you'll typically settle down for a larger meal and consequently more calories than you would normally eat per meal for three to six meals. Therefore, intermittent fasting is more about timing than the composition of your diet. Even then, you should avoid eating processed junk food, particularly those with empty calories since they will undo the benefits of your fast. Since intermittent fasting is more of a lifestyle, you'll do well to cut down on sweeteners and processed sugars and replace processed foods with whole foods. Ultimately, you should focus on having a balanced diet that includes whole grains, vegetables, fruits, and protein. If you're aiming at losing weight, you also must not take in too many calories during your feeding window.

Intermittent fasting helps you embrace a healthy lifestyle and avoid dangerous eating diets. Since intermittent fasting is not a diet, it's a lifestyle that can be sustained through the years. Intermittent fasting is more of a wellness revolution because it helps you to adapt to a lifestyle of eating healthy foods and avoiding dangerous diets. If you're on intermittent fasting, you should not overeat junk food; otherwise, you'll end up gaining weight. Remember, intermittent fasting isn't an excuse for indulging in your favorite chocolate cookie or ice cream without giving a care. Rather, intermittent fasting reprograms your brain so that you're accustomed to taking reduced calories than you would normally consume. This helps you to avoid the trap of overeating. In fact, you'll be surprised that over time you'll be able to say no to your favorite cookies not because you deny yourself a treat, but you simply don't want. When you're consuming fewer calories than you're taking, you'll definitely begin to burn fat and lose weight over time.

Intermittent fasting lets you have bigger meals that are more satisfying. When you have to eat every 2-3 hours, you tend to think about food for the better part of the day. Consequently, you'll hardly have big meals, particularly if you are physically inactive. Having infrequent meals in a large volume will often provide you with more calories and is much more satisfying hence a great way to feel fuller for longer periods. When you eat large meals infrequently, you'll have increased adherence to the diet over time.

Intermitted fasting helps to establish a more structured way of eating. When you are on the regular eating plan, you will, in most instances, find yourself snacking in between meals mindlessly. From a couple of cookies to a slice of cake and ice cream, there's always something you can chew on. This will definitely contribute to you gaining excess weight. Intermittent fasting helps you to structure your eating pattern without necessarily getting rid of your favorites. Instead, you eliminate the habit of eating every so often by taking better control of your diet.

Intermittent fasting improves your hunger awareness. Hunger and thirst are processed in the same part of the brain. Thus, it is common to find that you're eating throughout the day not because you're hungry but for other reasons. This can be anything from stress, boredom, happiness, or even sadness, among others. Sometimes, the mere smell of food can make you assume you're actually hungry. Thus, when you're on a fast, you'll have a heightened sense of hunger awareness that will make you realize that real hunger feels like and how to differentiate it from the hunger that is triggered by other factors.

You can still eat out and enjoy social gatherings during intermittent fasting. Unlike many weight loss diets, intermittent fasting is not restrictive in terms of the foods you need to include on your menu. So you don't have to worry about missing out on social gatherings or even eating out! In fact, this pattern of eating accommodates the social nature of human beings as we tend to build social events around food. Since most of the occasions take place in the evening, you can always stick to your fasting routine and join the rest of the gathering at the table. Intermittent fasting gives you the freedom to eat food that is served at social gatherings as well as restaurants while staying within your calorie range for the day. This makes it simple and easy to maintain. So you don't have to write off the idea of eating out.

You can still travel the world while fasting. If you love traveling, you might be hesitant about attempting intermittent fasting. However, the interesting thing is that you can still travel the world and not worry about missing new experiences because of breaking your fast outside your feeding window. You can easily integrate intermittent fasting into your diet so that you are enjoying new experiences while losing weight. This way, you don't have to eat unhealthy food or even abandon your intermittent fasting plan for weight loss. Intermittent fasting can work for you whenever and wherever you are.

Intermittent fasting helps to improve the quality of your sleep. Although most people embrace intermittent fasting solely to lose weight, it comes with other added benefits among them quality sleep. This is attributed to the fact that when you're fasting, your body digests food before you sleep. This eventually helps you to sleep better because your insulin and fat levels are better controlled. Getting quality sleep can also contribute to weight loss.

Intermittent fasting makes you feel happy. This is another added advantage of fasting for weight loss. When you lose excess weight, you will not only feel lighter but also happier because you'll be more confident in your body. Moreover, you'll also have more energy because generally, digestion often takes much of your body's energy. This is in addition to feeling more healthier and in control.

Intermittent fasting is easy to follow. In most cases, starting a diet is easy. However, many people tend to give up after several weeks of watching what you're eating and counting calories. On the contrary, intermittent fasting gives you much freedom making it a lot easier to stick with it in the long term.

Intermittent fasting helps in muscle growth. Although many people have reported that intermittent fasting resulted in the loss of muscle when done properly, intermittent fasting can contribute to muscle building. However, this will require you to tailor your intermittent fasting approach in a manner that limits your fasting period to between 10 and 12 hours so that you're not inhibiting the body's ability to build muscle. You may also have to extend your feeding window to 10 hours so that you get all the nutrients you need.

Well, intermittent fasting does more than just helping you achieve your goal of losing weight. It actually presents many other benefits that will generally improve your lifestyle. This means that you must stay committed to the intermittent fasting plan that works for you to make sure that you get the results you desire. Eventually, intermittent fasting will become part of your lifestyle.

Chapter 4: Impact of Intermittent Fasting on Your Body

A number of studies have backed up the fact that intermittent fasting presents powerful benefits to your brain and body. Some of the top benefits you'll experience when you embark on intermittent fasting for weight loss include the following:

Speeds up fat burning and weight loss. Intermittent fasting is one of the top strategies for burning fat effortlessly. Fat burning during intermittent fasting is actually a result of being in a calorie deficient state that promotes loss of fat. A study done on animals found that intermittent fasting for a period of up to 16 weeks helps in the preventions of obesity with the results being seen in just six weeks. According to researchers, intermittent fasting activates metabolism while also helping to burn more fat through the generation of body heat. When you're fasting, your insulin levels will be low. The body will break down carbohydrates into glucose that the cells will draw energy from or convert it into fat hence store it for later use. Insulin levels are low when you're not consuming food. Thus, during fasting, your insulin levels are likely to be low, prompting the cells to get their glucose from fat stores as energy. When this process is done repeatedly, it results in weight loss. Most research suggests that intermittent fasting may be an effective weight management strategy. The fact that you'll most likely be eating fewer calories than you're burning means that your body will mostly be relying on the fat stores for energy which will translate to significant weight loss.

Boosts growth hormone production. The physiology of fasting is interesting. As such, the power of fasting is not in the reduction of calories, but hormonal changes that take place. Fasting triggers increased the production of the human growth hormone (HGH) that is produced in the pituitary gland. This hormone is instrumental in the normal development in adolescents, children, and adults. In adults, a deficiency of the growth hormone results in an increase in body fat, a decrease in bone mass, and lower lean body mass. Upon release by the pituitary gland, the growth hormone lasts for just a few minutes in the bloodstream. This hormone goes to the liver for metabolism before conversion into various growth factors with the most important one being the Insulin-Like Growth Factor 1 (IGF1).

This Insulin-Like Growth Factor 1 is linked to high insulin levels as well as most poor health outcomes. Even then, the brief pulse of IGF1 from the human growth hormone only lasts for a few minutes. All hormones are secreted in brief bursts naturally ostensibly preventing the development of resistance that requires high levels as well as the persistence of those levels. This explains how insulin resistance develops. The human growth hormone is usually secreted during sleep as a counter-regulatory hormone. Together with adrenaline and cortisol, this the growth hormone increases your blood glucose by breaking down glycogen to counter insulin. These hormones are secreted in a pulse just before you wake up during a counter-regulatory surge. This is normal as it helps the ready prepare for the upcoming day.

It's, therefore, wrong to say that you derive the energy for the day from breakfast because usually, your body has already given a big shot for great stuff and fuel for the day. Therefore, you absolutely don't need to rely on all your sugary cereals for energy. This is also the reason why you least feel hungry in the morning even when you haven't eaten for 12 hours. The growth hormone tends to go down with age while abnormally low levels can result in low bone and muscle mass. Fasting stimulates the secretion of the human growth hormone. That is, when you fast, there's a spike in the morning and regular secretion throughout the day. This is critical to the maintenance of lean bone and muscle mass while the stored fats burn. When the growth hormone is elevated by fasting, your muscle mass increases.

Prevents insulin resistance. When you eat, the body breaks down the food into glucose that goes in the bloodstream for transportation to the cells. Your cells rely on this glucose as fuel to function properly. Insulin is a hormone that allows the cells to absorb glucose. Thus, whenever you eat insulin is produced, signaling the cells to absorb glucose. When the cells receive this glucose, they effectively receive energy. Even then, this is not always the case. In some instances, the communication between insulin and the cells can go off so that the glucose is not received in the cells but is instead stored as fat. This is referred to as insulin resistance. That is, as more and more insulin is produced, the cells do not respond by receiving glucose. Insulin resistance can be caused by various reasons, yet your pancreas can only produce so much insulin before it is fatigued, leading to insulin deficiency and subsequently, diabetes. When this happens, you'll constantly feel tired, cold, and lousy. This resistance is dependent on not only the levels of insulin but also the persistence level. Intermittent fasting is a great and easiest way of increasing your insulin sensitivity. When you burn the available glucose and glycogen that is the stored glucose, your body goes into ketosis where you draw energy from ketones.

Reduces the risk of heart disease. Heart disease is a leading killer across the world. CDC puts the number of people who die from heart disease in the United States at 610,000 annually. According to research, intermittent fasting can improve certain aspects of cardiovascular health. You can reduce the risk of heart disease by making changes to your lifestyle. This includes exercising, eating right, limiting your intake of alcohol, and not smoking. Intermittent fasting restricts the calories you consume on a given day it will improve your glycemic control, cardiovascular risk as well as insulin resistance. In one study, individuals who followed an alternate day fasting plan for successfully lost weight had a notable reduction in their blood sugar levels, inflammatory markers, blood pressure, triglycerides, LDL cholesterol, and the total cholesterol. Triglycerides are a type of fat that is found in the blood and is linked to heart disease.

Increases metabolic rate. Intermittent fasting helps in improving insulin sensitivity that is key in the prevention of diabetes, increasing metabolic rate, and weight management. It's a common belief that skipping meals will result in the body adapting to the calorie deficit by lowering the metabolic rate to save energy. It has been established that extended periods of fasting can lead to a drop in metabolism. However, some studies have also shown that when you fast for short periods, you can increase your metabolism. In fact, one study conducted among 11 healthy men found that after a three day fast, their metabolism actually increased by 14%. This increase is attributed to the rise in norepinephrine hormone that, together with insulin, promotes fat burning. Based on these findings, intermittent fasting is far much significant with great weight loss advantages when compared to the other diets that are aimed to focus on calorie restriction for losing weight. Even then, the effects of intermittent fasting on metabolism are still under study because several other studies have found that your muscle mass doesn't decrease much during intermittent fasting.

Intermittent fasting changes how cells, genes, and hormones function. There's a raft of activities that go on in your body when you fast for extended periods. One of the things that happens is that your body will initiate important cellular repair processes as well as a change in the levels of hormones to make stored fat more accessible. More specifically, there'll be a significant drop in the insulin levels resulting in fat burning as the stored fats become a primary source of energy. The growth hormone in the blood may increase up to five times that also facilitates fat burning and muscle gain. Fasting also results in beneficial changes, molecules, and genes that are related to protection against disease and longevity. Cellular repair processes are also initiated when you're fasting promoting the removal of waste material from the cells.

Reduces inflammation and oxidative stress in the body. Oxidative stress is a step in most of the chronic diseases and aging. It involves unstable molecules known as free radicals that react with other molecules like DNA and protein and damage them. A number of studies show that intermittent fasting enhances your body's resistance to oxidative stress. In addition, intermittent fasting also helps in fighting inflammation that is a common cause of diseases, especially when your body is able to go into autophagy.

Induces a number of cellular repair processes. When you fast for extended periods, the cells in your body begin to initiate a waste removal process that is known as autophagy. This process not only involves breaking down but also metabolizing dysfunctional and broken proteins that accumulate in within the cells over time. Increased autophagy is able to offer protection against a number of diseases such as Alzheimer's disease.

Helps in the prevention of cancer. Cancer is a disease that is characterized by the growth of cells that is uncontrolled. Studies have found that fasting has a number of benefits on metabolism that could actually lead to a reduced risk of cancer. There's also evidence on cancer patients showing that fasting reduced some of the side effects of chemotherapy. It's important to note that these studies have mostly been done in animals; hence, there's a need for further studies in humans.

Fasting has anti-aging effects. Various forms of fasting have been found to improve healthspan and lifespan significantly. This has been demonstrated with caloric restriction in animals that reduces the number of calories by between 20 and 30%. Intermittent fasting also slows down the aging process and increases your lifespan by manipulating mitochondrial networks. Mitochondria are power generators found in the cells. They produce most of the energy the cells need for survival. Studies have shown that intermittent fasting helps to keep the mitochondrial networks fused hence keeping the mitochondria strong with the ability to process energy. This is crucial for vibrant aging and longevity. Fasting also delays the aging process and prevent diseases by triggering adaptive cellular stress responses that result in a better ability to cope with more stress while counteracting the disease. Thus, when your mitochondria work better, so will your body.

Intermittent fasting is therapeutic. When practiced well, intermittent fasting offers therapeutic benefits that are psychological, spiritual, and physical. For physical benefits, intermittent fasting can help cure diabetes. In addition, it has been proven to be extremely useful in the reduction of seizure-related brain damage as well as seizures themselves as well as improve symptoms of arthritis. Fasting also offers spiritual benefits, as is widely practiced by different religions around the world. It contributes towards purifying your soul and body when practiced within the religious context. The psychological angle of fasting is in the fact that it takes your will and self-control, which is a powerful psychological benefit. You learn how to ignore hunger and practice restraint from eating for a certain duration. This is a great practice because it's about training your mind. A successful intermittent fasting plan will have powerful effects on your psychological perspective. In fact, intermittent fasting has been proven to have positive results in women, especially in relation to improving the sense of control, pride, achievement, and reward. Moreover, it is handy for improving your self-esteem.

You need to understand how intermittent fasting will affect you before you get into it because this signals a change of lifestyle. While it may seem difficult to execute because your body is used to a certain way of eating, it's doable, and the results are incredible. The only thing you should never do is wake up one morning and jump into it. Rather, take time to prepare psychologically and begin slowly to increase your success rate, especially if you're looking to embrace healthy living by making a lifestyle change.

Chapter 5: Benefits of Intermittent Fasting

You've probably been told to make sure that you eat a balanced diet. Thus, it's odd to think that depriving yourself a meal or more can actually be a necessity. Interestingly, evidence points to the benefits of intermittent fasting on your wellbeing. Different forms of intermittent fasting will yield different benefits that go beyond weight loss. Some of the benefits of intermittent fasting include:

Weight and body fat loss. The majority of people who try intermittent fasting do it because they want to lose weight. Unlike other weight loss plan, intermittent fasting makes you adapt to an eating pattern that defines when you should eat and when you should fast. The whole idea behind intermittent fasting it offers you flexibility while making you eat fewer meals. This is not equivalent to counting calories as is usually the norm with most of the weight loss regimens. When you alter your eating pattern, then you're likely to eat much less hence taking fewer calories. In addition, intermittent fasting will enhance the hormonal function that facilitates weight loss. That is, a dip in the levels of insulin, along with a higher presence of the growth hormone and an increase in the amount of norepinephrine increases the rate at which fat is broken down into energy. As such, fasting on a short-term basis will increase your metabolic rate, thus helping you to burn more fats. Thus, intermittent fasting works to lose weight by reducing the amount of food you eat as well as boost your metabolic rate. It's estimated that you can experience up to 8% weight loss over a period of 3-24 weeks with intermittent fasting. When you have significant weight loss, your waist circumference will also reduce indicating loss of belly fat that is actually harmful.

Stable glucose level. Studies conducted in both people and mice show that various kinds of intermittent fasting can improve the way your body responds to sugar. In mice, researchers were able to reboot the pancreas that produces insulin, thereby reversing diabetes. Various forms of fasting that involve extended hours of unrestricted eating, followed by five days of eating a restricted fasting diet has been found to cause big improvements in individuals with high blood sugar. Losing weight, eating healthy, and moving more can help in fighting off the development of type 2 diabetes. Losing weight makes you more insulin sensitive hence driving your blood sugar down. When you eat, your body releases insulin in your bloodstream to supply cells energy. However, if you're pre-diabetic, your insulin resistant meaning your blood sugar levels are constantly elevated. Thus intermittent fasting can help to stabilize your glucose levels since it requires your body to produce insulin less often hence restoring your insulin secretion and promoting the generation of new insulin-producing pancreatic beta cells according to research.

Improves digestive health. The cells with the gastrointestinal tract are constantly working. In some instances, these cells work to the extent of being passed out a part of excreta. You can repair these digestive cells with intermittent fasting by making sure your body gets to autophagy. This gets rid of the old cells and activates your immune system accordingly. This also applies to a chronic gut immune response that is capable of inflaming bowels. Getting them to rest allows them a chance to restore and repair. An extended night fast and autophagy will give your gut a chance not only to relax but also recharge.

Improved brain health. Studies conducted in mice show that intermittent fasting could actually improve brain health by boosting your brainpower. As you grow older, the amount of blood flowing to your brain decreases while the neurons shrink, and the brain volume declines. Intermittent fasting halts the aging process keeping you mentally healthy and sharp. By boosting your brain health, intermittent fasting can lower your risk of neurodegenerative diseases like Parkinson's and Alzheimer's.

Furthermore, fasting reduces obesity and is able to protect you from diabetes, both of which can increase your risk of developing Alzheimer's disease. Intermittent fasting also helps in improving your brain by hindering the degeneration of nerve cells. According to one study, intermittent fasting plays an important role in guarding neurons in the brain from excitotoxic stress. In addition, it also speeds up autophagy in the neurons helping your body to eliminate all the damaged cells while generating new ones. This is important in helping the body defend itself from diseases. Your memory and learning ability also improve with intermittent fasting. Studies have shown that memory and mood are boosted after periods of caloric restriction.

Decreased risk of cancer. Cancer has become prevalent over the past few years, affecting people of all ages and race. The good news is that autophagy promises to reduce the likelihood of having cancer. Autophagy has received attention from medical professionals for its role in the prevention of cancer. This is because cancer occurs when there's a cellular disorder thus by promoting cell inflammation as well as regulation of damage response to the DNA by foreign bodies and regulating genome instability it helps to keep cancer at bay.

Promotes longevity. Intermittent fasting can help promote the overall length of life. This concept dates back to the 1950s when scientists discovered autophagy as well as the great potential it holds in determining the quality of life. That is, you don't necessarily need to take in too many nutrients to ensure your wellbeing rather, work toward promoting the internal process that recycles the damaged cell parts and eliminates the toxic body cells.

Improve immune system. Autophagy is powerful and highly effective when it comes to keeping your immune system in top shape. It achieves this by promoting inflammation in cells as well as actively fighting diseases through non-selective autophagy. When cellular inflammation happens, it boosts the cells of the immune system whenever it is attacked by diseases. Autophagy induces inflammation by depriving cell proteins of nutrition, thereby causing them to work more actively. This initiates the required immune response that keeps diseases and infections away. It also eliminates harmful elements that include tuberculosis, micro bacterium, as well as other viral elements from the cell.

Regulates inflammation. You can either reduce or boost the immune response with autophagy depending on what is required. This, in turn, prevents and promotes inflammation. When there's a dangerous invasion, autophagy will boost inflammation by signaling the immune system to attack. On the other hand, it can also decrease the inflammation within the immune system by getting rid of the signals that cause it.

Improved quality of life. The internet is awash with tons of methods and techniques that guarantee quality health and quality life in general. The truth is that none of these methods that include diets, anti-aging creams, and other products can lead closer to autophagy during intermittent fasting. The cellular degeneration and regeneration processes during autophagy are guaranteed to make you appear youthful in contrast to your actual age. This is especially important to your skin that is exposed to harsh elements of pollution as well as other substance that cause wrinkles leading to a decline in your skin quality with layers of toxic substances forming over your skin cells.

Decreased risk of neurodegenerative diseases. When your body achieves autophagy, you'll have a decreased risk of developing neurodegenerative diseases like Alzheimer's and Parkinson's. Here's how. Neurodegenerative diseases will work well on the basis of the accumulated toxic and old neurons that pile up in certain areas of the brain spreading to the surrounding areas. Therefore, autophagy replaces the neuron parts that are useless and, in their place, regenerate new ones effectively keeping these diseases in check.

Enhanced mental performance. Intermittent fasting enhances the cognitive function in addition to being useful in boosting brain power. Intermittent fasting will boost the brain-derived neurotrophic factor (BDNF) levels. This is a protein within the brain that is able to interact with the other parts of your brain that are responsible for controlling the learning, memory, and cognitive functions. The brain-derived neurotrophic factor is also capable of protecting and stimulating the growth of new brain cells. When you are on intermittent fasting, your body will go into the ketogenic state, thereby using ketones to burn body fat to energy. Ketones are also capable of feeding your brain, thus improving your mental productivity, energy, and acuity.

Prevention of diseases. Intermittent fasting has been associated with the prevention of diseases. According to research, intermittent fasting plays an important role in improving the number of risk markers for chronic disease that include lowered cholesterol, lowered blood pressure, and reduced insulin resistance. A study in the World Journal of Diabetes reveals that patients who have type 2 diabetes and are on short term daily intermittent fasting are likely to experience a drop in their lower body weight and have better variability of post-meal glucose. Intermittent fasting will also enhance stress markers resistance, reduce inflammation and blood pressure and promote better glucose circulation and lipid levels hence reducing the risk of cardiovascular diseases such as cancer, Alzheimer's, and Parkinson's. Intermittent fasting can also slow down the progression of certain cancers like skin and breast cancer by increasing the levels of tumor-infiltrating lymphocytes. These are the cells that are sent by the immune system to attack the tumor.

Improved physical fitness. Intermittent fasting influences your digestive system; hence, your level of physical fitness. Having a small feasting window and an extended fasting window encourages proper digestion of food. As a result, you have a healthy and proportional daily intake of food as well as calories. As you get used to this process, it is unlikely that you will experience hunger. You don't have to worry about slowing down your metabolism because, in reality, intermittent fasting will enhance your metabolism making it more flexible as your body has the capability to run on fats and glucose along for energy effectively. The use of oxygen is important in the success of your training. In fact, in order to perform well, you must adjust your breathing habits during workouts. Generally, the maximum amount of oxygen that your body uses per kilogram of your body weight or per minute is referred to as VO2. This is also known as wind. The amount of wind you have influences your performance. More wind means better performance.

Consequently, top athletes will have twice as much VO2 level compared to those without training. A study carried out on a fasted group that skipped breakfast and a non-fasted group that had breakfast an hour before found that the VO2 levels of both groups were 3.5L/min at the beginning. There was a notable increase in the wind in the fasting group at 9.7% compared to an increase of 2.5% in those who took breakfast.

Enhances bodybuilding. When you have a short feasting window, it automatically translates to fewer meals meaning you can concentrate your daily intake of calories in 1-2 meals. Bodybuilders find this approach to be great compared to splitting your calories in 5-6 meals spread throughout the day. You need a certain amount of protein in maintaining your muscle mass. You can still maintain your muscle mass with intermittent fasting even though this eating pattern doesn't focus on your protein intake. Since your growth hormone reaches unbelievable levels after 48 hours of fasting, you're able to maintain muscles even without having to eat proteins or even having protein shakes and bars.

Increased insulin sensitivity. Insulin sensitivity refers to your body cell's level of sensitivity in response to insulin. High levels of insulin sensitivity are good as it allows the cells to use blood glucose effectively, thereby reducing the amount of blood sugar in your system. When your insulin levels are low, you will experience insulin resistance. When this happens, you will experience abnormal levels of blood sugar, which, when not managed, will result in type 2 diabetes. Insulin sensitivity will vary between different people and will change according to various dietary factors and lifestyle. Therefore, improving it could be beneficial to those people who are living with or are at risk of developing type 2 diabetes. According to a 2014 review investigating the effect of intermittent fasting in obese and overweight adults, intermittent fasting has the ability to reduce insulin resistance. Even then, there was no significant effect on glucose levels.

Intermittent fasting will provide amazing results when done right. From the loss of excessive weight to a reversal of type 2 diabetes, many benefits are linked to intermittent fasting. Even then, you need to stay committed and be consistent with your intermittent fasting protocol in order to achieve results. Most importantly, make sure you have a goal you'd like to achieve at the beginning of your fasting period. While at it remember that unlike many weight loss diets, fasting doesn't have a standard duration because it's just about depriving your body food for a given time.

Intermittent fasting is nothing curious or queer rather; it's part of normal everyday life. It's the most powerful and oldest intervention you can think of, yet so many people are not aware of its power to rejuvenate the body as well as its therapeutic potential. You don't have to put pressure on yourself to produce results in the beginning, especially if your goal is to lose weight. Take time to transition, allowing your body to adjust accordingly. This may mean starting with a plan that is close to your current eating plan, slowly advancing to intermittent eating plans that require you to fast for longer durations.

Chapter 6: Intermittent Fasting: The Best Anti-Aging Diet

Countless celebrities and entrepreneurs use intermittent fasting to reverses the effects of aging. However, not everyone understands the scientific aspect of intermittent fasting and its link with anti-aging. This chapter looks into the scientific aspect of intermittent fasting while introducing concepts related to aging healthily. To understand the relationship between fasting and anti-aging, you first need to understand the difference between the various fasting methods. For starters, the short-term fasting plans with a fasting window of between 16 and 20 hours offer multiple independent benefits. These fasts that are also known as micro-fasts support metabolic healthy by controlling body weight, lowering your insulin levels, and improving glycemic control. As such, short term fasting is an incredible choice to embrace when your goal is solely weight loss. During short fasts, your fat mass may reduce while physical strength remains the same.

The other benefits of fasting include an increase in brain-derived neurotrophic factor (BDNF) signaling within your brain, cardiovascular support, and reduced risk of cancer recurrence. On the other hand, fasting for extended periods will stimulate physiological changes that offer unique benefits of fasting that fall within functional areas like longevity, immune strength, and healthy aging.

The physiological effects of extended fasting are more pronounced than the effects of short-term fasts lasting less than 24 hours because of the body's ability to switch to fat and ketone catabolism upon the depletion of glycogen reserves during extended fasting. Extended fasting also increased the white blood cells that are a biomarker for immune health and is useful for adjunct therapy alongside chemotherapy for killing cancer cells. The rationale behind this is that cancer cells grow and thrive on glucose; thus, when you go on extended fasts; you starve the cancer cells and support the anti-cancer immune efforts.

Anti-Aging Benefits of Intermitted Fasting

Out of all interventions that are aimed at countering aging, calorie restriction is that most efficient. Generally, fasting for extended periods results in calorie restriction that reduces calories by between 20 and 40%. This is not recommended for performance and is unpopular among biohackers owing to mental distraction. Calorie restriction promotes five mechanisms that are essential for healthy aging. The following are mechanisms of extended fasting that promote healthy aging.

These processes are:

Cell proliferation (IGF-1 and TOR; specifically mTOR): Cell proliferation promotes balanced cell growth. It is the ability of the human system to be in the anabolic state with the presence of calories. That is, whenever calories are abundant, cells are in an anabolic state. When you're intermittent fasting results in caloric restriction that tends to shift the balance in the system through stimulation of catabolic pathways. The two pathways that are important in this process are the mammalian target of rapamycin (mTOR) and insulin-like growth factor-1 (IGF-1). Both IGF-1 and mTOR are nutrient sensors that regulate the cellular resources depending on the availability of calories. When you fast, fewer calories are leading to the down-regulation of mTOR and IGF-1, thus signaling repurposing and recycling of organelles and cells. A decline in mTOR signaling has been found to lead to lifespan extension.

Moreover, its inhibition is known to be a longevity assurance mechanism with the availability of rapamycin as well as other mTOR inhibitors making this pathway a valuable target for interventions that extend lifespan. Dr. Jason Fung, a proponent of intermittent fasting, agrees that mTOR is a protein sensor. He further says that eating fats alone and no protein can theoretically modulate MTOR positively. Thus, you can include fat-based drinks in your micro-fast.

Decreased Inflammation (NF-kB): The human body is bound to experience cumulative damage as you age. The damage is often identified by the immune receptors, thereby stimulating the production of multiple proinflammatory molecules. In the worst-case scenario, the accumulated damage is so extensive that the inflammation becomes continuous that either accompanies numerous age-related diseases or contributes to them. Inflammation on its own is not necessarily bad since its part of healing. However, evidence suggests that chronic inflammation and specifically age-associated inflammation, also referred to inflaming, heavily correlates with poor health biomarkers. Calorie restriction during intermittent fasting will inhibit nuclear factor kB (NF-kB) that exerts the anti-inflammatory effect. NF-kB is believed to the master regulator of inflammation, thus minimizing its activity will downregulate various parts of the proinflammatory signaling. Animal models suggest that this anti-inflammatory effect may have cognitive enhancing properties. One study focused on fasting as eustress; a form of stress that is beneficial versus distress; the negative stressors of life that speed up aging. The conclusion was that intermittent fasting led to a reduction of the plasma inflammatory factors. Thus, intermittent fasting can improve cognitive function and preserve the brain from distress through regulation of inflammatory response pathway. By engaging in intermittent fasting, you're able to attain the beneficial levels of stress that is necessary for your physiology and psychology.

Improved mitochondrial physiology (AMPK/SIRT): Mitochondria are the organelles that make up a cell. They're crucial in the production of cellular energy that enables the cells to do more work. This work is equivalent to physical labor, as is the case with the muscle cells or cognitive tasks in the case of brain cells. Aging tends to weaken the general quality of your body's mitochondrial network, thereby decreasing the destruction of already damaged or dysfunctional mitochondria as well as the generation of new mitochondria. However, when you fast and experience calorie restriction, these processes will be supported, giving rise to a high quality of your mitochondrial network. The two pathways that are mostly associated with mitochondrial support are sirtuins (SIRT genes) and AMP-dependent kinase (AMPK). Both pathways are sensitive to the shifts in the NADH/NAD+ ratio. Calorie restriction triggers an increase in NAD+ accumulation that activates sirtuins and AMPK. Studies have concluded that the fact that sirtuins need NAD for their enzymatic activity links metabolism to diseases associated with aging and aging. Both sirtuins and AMPK are central to mitochondrial biogenesis as well as processes of mitophagy (mitochondrial removing and recycling of the organelles that are dysfunctional that are associated with age) are important in maintaining a younger mitochondrial network. When cells are deprived of glucose during an extended fast, the production of ATP initially drops. When AMPK senses the decrease in ATP, it limits the utilization of energy as it upregulates numerous other processes that replenish ATP. As a result, mitochondria and cells are able to better make ATP in the future. Calorie restriction activates the AMPK pathway in a number of tissues in animal models. However, this has not been studied in humans. Sirtuins also play an important role in aging as a biological stress sensor. Increasing and manipulating the expression of sirtuins in yeast promotes longevity.

Enhanced autophagy (FoxO): Autophagy can loosely be translated to self-eating. That is a cleaning mechanism that involves removal of organelles, old cell membranes as well as other cellular junk that has accumulated with time and is an impediment to optimal cellular performance. When the old and broken parts of your cells are removed, the growth hormone that is usually amplified during fasting will signal the body to start the production of new replacements. The result of autophagy is the renovation and recycling process of cells. mTOR will induce the activation of the forkhead box proteins. Both mitophagy and autophagy are FoxO-dependent suggesting that the transcriptional molecule is an integral component of the processes.

Increased antioxidant defenses (Nrf2): As humans age, there's an increase in the reactive oxygen species (ROS) while the natural antioxidant defenses decrease. Over time, this imbalance becomes greater even as the damage accumulates while the mitochondrial dysfunction becomes more prevalent. The normal production of oxidants in specific types of cells is important in the regulation of pathways (ROS are involved in some of the signaling processes). Therefore, it is valuable to strike the right balance as we age. This balance is may be critical for the optimization of mitochondrial performance and is referred to as mitohormesis with the idea being the need for the right amount of ROS with too little resulting in subpar performance while high amounts of ROS cause damage. This is important for those tissues that rely on the production of large amounts of ATP for metabolism such as heart, brain, and muscle. Among the understandings from mitorhormesis is that a certain amount of ROS is required to trigger adaptive responses that upregulate the antioxidant defenses as well as make mitochondria and cells better in dealing with toxins and stress. Thus, intermittent fasting can help in promoting anti-oxidant defenses. Calorie restriction will activate the nuclear factor (erythroid-derived 2) like 2 (Nfr2) that is a regulator of the cellular resistance to the oxidants. This protein plays a role in supporting antioxidant defenses through:

- Catabolism of peroxides and superoxide; eliminating all the bad stuff.
- Regeneration of oxidized proteins and cofactors (regrowing more of the good old stuff)
- Increase of redox transport (increasing efficiency of existing machinery)
- Synthesis of reducing factors (Creation of new good stuff)

Overall, Nrf2 is not the only mechanisms that promote antioxidant support and defenses. All the five mechanisms that are interrelated owing to the complex nature of human systems contribute to healthspan longevity. Like it is with all these other mechanisms, they support each other. For instance, mTOR is not only categorized under cell proliferation and autophagy.

Intermittent Fasting for Lifespan and Healthspan

Lifespan refers to the duration of time that you've lived. On the other hand, the duration within which you've been functional and healthy, and not just being alive is referred to as the healthspan. Calorie restriction that is initiated by any form of intermittent fasting is important in affecting both your lifespan and healthspan. It's not unusual to focus on the lifespan within the longevity and aging space at the expense of the quality of life you're living.

On the contrary, the duration of time you're functional and healthy is correlated with a higher quality of life. Your healthspan can be mediated by many things among them; dietary interventions, social interactions, exercise, family, and community. Social interaction is positively related to life satisfaction and longevity. Thus, healthspan it may be more valuable to emphasize lifespan alone.

Damage Accumulation vs. Programmed Aging

The debate between the importance of damage accumulation and programmed aging is unending. Humans are complex systems that involve a combination of both. Damage accumulation is characterized by mitochondrial and cellular damage, both of which happen at the cellular level with each amplifying the effects of the other. That is the changes in gene expression speed up damage accumulation, which in turn affects the ability of the cell to have healthy gene expression. On the other hand, programmed aging refers to changes in the manner in which our genes are expressed as we age. Some of the genes are underexpressed, while others are overexpressed.

Aging Benefits of Intermittent Fasting

The scientific aspect of the mechanisms that are involved in promoting longevity and aging go beyond the context of fasting. These mechanisms determine nootropics as well as the other techniques that we can use in supporting healthy aging. Although there are many benefits that arise when a certain degree of temporary starvation is induced, it's important to note that there are more ways to trigger these responses. Most importantly, you need to keep in mind that while some of the benefits will occur while you're in the fasted state, others will happen when you start eating normally. Thus, starvation primes the systems for rejuvenation even though it is refeeding that is credited for rebuilding new organelles and cells, thus increasing health.

Intermittent Fasting and Anti-aging Compounds

Excessive levels of pyrimidine and purine are signs that your body might be experiencing an increase in the levels of certain antioxidants. Specifically, researchers have found significant increases in carnosine and ergothioneine. A study on the individual variability in human blood metabolites found that the number of metabolites decreases as you age. These metabolites include ophthalmic acid, isoleucine, and leucine. This study also found that fasting significantly boosted the three metabolites and concluded that this explains how fasting extends the lifespan in rats. It is believed that the hike in antioxidants may be a survival response because when in the fasted state, the body experiences extreme levels of oxidative stress. Thus, the production of antioxidants can help in avoiding the potential damage that is a result of free radicals.

Intermittent Fasting and the Anti-Aging Molecule

Research has found that being in the fasted state is instrumental in triggering a molecule that can cause a delay in the aging of arteries. This is important in the prevention of chronic diseases that are age-related like cardiovascular disease, cancer, and Alzheimer's and is evidence that aging can be reversed. Vascular aging is the most important aspect of aging. Thus, when people grow older, they vessels supplying blood to various organs become more sensitive and more likely to experience aging damage; thus studying is vascular aging is important. According to the research done on starving mice generated a molecule known as beta-hydroxybutyrate that prevented vascular aging. This molecule is also a ketone that is produced by the liver and is handy as an energy source; then the glucose level is low. Ketones are mostly produced during starvation or fasting or when you're on a diet comprising low carbs and after a prolonged exercise. This molecule also promotes the multiplication and division of cells lining the blood vessels. This is a market of cellular youth.

Additionally, this compound is also able to delay vascular aging through endothelial cells that line lymphatic vessels and blood vessels. This can prevent the kind of cell aging that is referred to as cellular aging or senescence. Cellular senescence is defined as the irreversible cell cycle while at the same time preserving the cellular viability. Cellular senescence is suggested to work as a tumor suppressor mechanism as well as tissue remodeling promoter after wounding. These cells show marked changes in morphology that includes irregular shape size, enlarged size, multiple and prominent nuclei, increased granularity, accumulation of lysosomal, and mitochondrial mass.

Chapter 7: The Golden Key: Autophagy

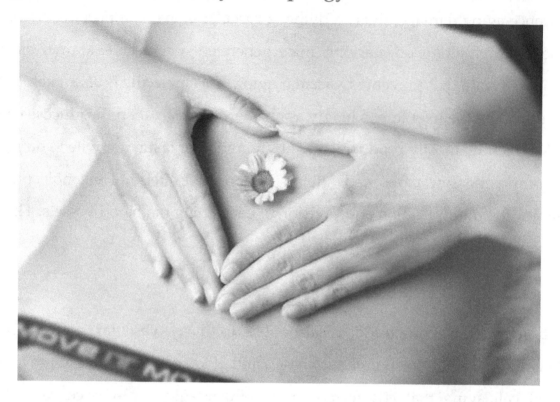

The cells in the human body are constantly being damaged as metabolic processes take place hence the need for autophagy to clear these damaged cells. The word autophagy comes from two Greek words; 'auto' which means self and 'phagy' meaning eating. Thus, autophagy is the process where the body consumes its own tissue in the wake of metabolic processes that occur due to certain diseases and starvation. Researchers consider autophagy to be a survival mechanism or the body's clever way of responding to stress to protect itself.

When you think of it as a form of self-eating, it's definitely scary. So is autophagy good for your health? Definitely! This is the body's normal way of initiating the process of cellular renewal. Autophagy may seem like a relatively new concept, yet our bodies have been using it for millions of years. The first autophagy studies were conducted on yeast with the progress of this study leading to a Nobel Prize in

Physiology or Medicine for Dr. Yoshinori Ohsumi, a Japanese scientist for his discoveries of the mechanisms of autophagy in October 2016. According to the study, the body can eliminate all the clutter within whenever it feels the need to conserve the energy for other most important purposes. The cleaning mechanism of autophagy is critical in the elimination of just about every kind of toxins, misfolded proteins, germs, bacteria, and pathogens. So beneficial is autophagy that is key in preventing diseases like liver disease, cancer, infections, diabetes, cardiomyopathy, neurodegeneration, autoimmune diseases. Autophagy offers multiple anti-aging benefits by helping in destroying and reusing damaged components that occur within cells. Thus, this process uses the waste generated within cells to create new building materials that facilitate regeneration and repair. Although the process of autophagy doesn't require any outside help, you'll definitely begin feeling more relaxed and energetic once it takes place.

While recent studies have revealed the role of autophagy in cleaning and defending the body from the negative effects of stress, the exact way autophagy processes work is just beginning to be understood. Several processes are involved. For instance, lysosomes form part of the cells that are capable of destroying large damages cells such as mitochondria as well as help in transporting the damaged parts, so they are used to generate fuel. To sum it up, the damaged material must be transported by a lysosome, before it's deconstructed and spit back out for repurposing.

Essential Autophagy Steps

The process of autophagy involves the following steps as follows:

1. Creation of phagophore by a protein kinase complex as well as a lipid kinase complex. These two work together in sourcing a membrane that will eventually become the phagophore.

2. Once the phagophore is formed, the next step is its expansion. In this stage, a protein that is known as LC3 is bonded with the just formed phogophore through multiple autophagy-related proteins that are referred to as the ATG. When the bonding of the two is complete, the LC3 protein then becomes LC3-II. This formation occurs around cytoplasm material, which is then due to be degraded. This material may be random or selected specifically if it includes misfolded proteins and damaged organelles. When the process of replacement begins, ATG-9, a transmembrane protein acting as a protector of the site of phagophore formation is formed. This protein is assumed to help in expansion by increasing the number of phagophore membrane by supplying them from adjacent membrane locations.

3. The phagophore undergoes changes in its shape becoming elongated and closing, thereby becoming an autophagosome. The autophagosome serves as a holder of materials that are then degraded.

4. Both lysosome and autophagosome membranes fuse together. The lysosomal lumen (space within a lysosome) have hydrolases. Hydrolases break down molecules into smaller pieces using water to demolish the chemical bonds. When the lysosome and autophagosome fuse together, an exposure of the material that is inside the autophagosome to chemical wrecking balls occurs. The fusion converts the lysosome into an autolysosome.

5. The hydrolases degrade all material found within the autophagosome together with the inner membrane. The macromolecules that are the result of this process are waddled around by permeases that are on the autolysosome membrane until they get back to their original cytoplasm. At this point, the cell may reuse the macromolecules.

Well, this is how autophagy works. It's a complex yet important process that is still being studied to ensure further understanding.

There are different kinds of autophagy that include micro and macroautophagy as well as chaperone-mediated autophagy. Macroautophagy is the most popular of the three. It is an evolutionarily conserved anabolic process that involves the formation of autophagosomes (vesicles) that surround cellular organelles and macromolecules. Apart from humans' mold, yeast, flies, worms, and mammals also benefit from autophagy.

Macroautophagy is the process where catalyzation of non-functional cellular constituents to lysosome of cells takes place. What this process does is a separation of the cytoplasm of cells that includes different cell organs, degrading them to amino acids.

Inducing Autophagy With Intermittent Fasting

One of the common questions about autophagy is when does it occur? Generally, autophagy is usually active in all the cells. However, there's increased response to acute energy shortage, nutrient deprivation, and stress. This means that you can cause your body to go into autophagy using good stressors such as temporary calorie restriction and exercise. These have been linked with longevity, weight control as well as inhibiting a number of age-related diseases.

You can induce autophagy through intermittent fasting. When you restrain yourself from eating food for a while, it will eventually trigger autophagy. When you fast for long, your body will start feeling deprived of supply hence can begin catabolic processes at the macromolecular level. This means identifying those processes that are misusing the available energy like parasites, pathogens, mold, fungi, and bacteria within that don't give back anything for elimination. Once your body goes into autophagy, it begins the elimination by identifying all misfolded proteins and recycling them to produce energy and new cells. Not only does this process clean your body but also promote restrengthening. The body also identifies chronic inflammations, disorders, and diseases that make us ill and use the energy of the body and eliminates them. When the elimination begins, even chronic inflammations that have troubled you for years will go away, making autophagy a powerful mechanism of treatment. This also has a powerful anti-aging effect because it stops those processes that hasten the signs of aging. Autophagy also has a great impact on the cognitive function in addition to stopping neurodegenerative disorders and reversing their effects. This means that disorders like Parkinson's and Alzheimer's can be brought under control. Autophagy also promotes cardiovascular health, lowers immunity problems, hypertension, and chronic inflammation. This process is guaranteed to give you a boon for a rejuvenated life.

Studies suggest that the autophagy process starts anywhere between 24 and 48 hours after your last meal. This is perhaps one of the best ways of inducing autophagy. Therefore, if you would like to trigger autophagy, then you must fast for longer. Alternate day fasting and water fasting are the most ideal. If you opt for alternate day fasting, make sure that you don't eat anything during the 36-hour fasting window. Don't consume any calories from soft drinks or juices either. On the other hand, if you go for the water fast, you must do it for 2 to 3 days as your recommended fasting window of between 24 to 48 hours.

Ultimately, the best intermittent fasting you can employ to induce autophagy is alternate day fast without consuming any calories in the fasting window. If you feel you're up to it, you can take it a notch higher with a 2- t0 3-day water fast once in three months. Looking at the benefits, it's definitely worth restraining yourself from eating to get your body into autophagy.

Exercise is another source of good stress that has been found to induce autophagy. According to recent research, exercise induces autophagy in a number of organs that take part in metabolic regulation like liver, muscle, adipose tissue, and pancreas. Although exercise has many benefits to the body, it's a form of stress since it breaks down tissues and causes them to be repaired so that they grow back stronger. Although the extent of exercise required to boost autophagy is not clear, research suggests that going into intense exercise is most beneficial. If you want to combine fasting and exercise, then you must approach it with caution. You just might be surprised that you actually feel energetic once you get the hang of fasting.

Apart from fasting and exercise, there are certain foods which, when eaten, will contribute towards inducing autophagy. Generally speaking, you need to focus on low carb foods, some of which include the following:

Herbs and spices such as cayenne pepper, black pepper, ginseng, ginger, cinnamon, turmeric, cumin, cardamom, parsley, thyme, cilantro, coriander, rosemary, and basil.

Berries and other fruits; strawberries, raspberries, blueberries, elderberries, cherries and cranberries.

Drinks; tea and coffee. Your coffee and tea should have no cream, milk, or sugar. As such, it's better to go for herbal, green, or black tea. Avoid fruit tea since it's too sweet. You may also have distilled vinegar or apple cider.

Alcoholic drinks; vodka, vermouth, gin, whiter, and red wine.

You could also try foods that are healthy for your body that include the following:

Fruits such as; olive, avocado, coconut, watermelon, cantaloupe, and honeydew.

Veggies; squash, tomato, peas, spinach, bell pepper, pickles, beetroot, green beans, carrots, and turnip.

Seeds and nuts; brazil nuts, almonds, cashews, chia seeds, chestnuts, flax seeds, macadamia, hazelnuts, pecans, peanuts, pistachios, pine nuts, pumpkin seeds, sunflower, sesame seeds, walnuts, peanut butter, almond butter, cashew butter, and macadamia nut butter.

Dairy and milk; blue cheese, buttermilk, brie cheese, Colby cheese, cheddar cheese, cottage cheese, cream cheese, Monterey jack cheese, mozzarella, feta cheese, swiss cheese, parmesan, mascarpone, sour cream, heavy cream, skimmed milk, and whole milk.

Fats; coconut milk, coconut cream, red palm oil, olive oil, MCT oil, macadamia oil, flaxseed oil, coconut oil, cocoa butter, avocado oil, beef tallow, lard, lard, ghee and butter.

Protein shakes with water; whey protein shake, hemp protein shake, rice protein shake, pea protein shake, and microgreens blend.

Drinks; almond water, almond milk, coconut water, kombucha, and coconut milk.

Alcoholic drinks; cognac, tequila, champagne, beer, mint liquor and chocolate liquor.

There's more to learn about autophagy and the best way of inducing it. Combing fasting and regular exercise as part of your daily routine is a great place to start. If you're taking certain medications for any health condition, you must consult your doctor before you go into fasting.

Uses of Autophagy

The main function of autophagy is degrading and breaking down organelles in cells. This process contributes to the repair of cells. Autophagy also acts as part of the body's repair mechanism. Autophagy also plays an important role in a number of cellular functions like yeast the high levels of autophagy are activated by nutrient starvation. In addition to degrading unnecessary proteins, autophagy is also helpful in recycling amino acids that in turn, are important in synthesizing proteins that are crucial for survival. In the case of animals, they experience nutrient depletion after birth due to severing transplacental food supply. It is at this point that autophagy is activates helping to mediate the nutrient depletion. Another function of autophagy is xenophagy, which is the breaking down of the infectious particles.

Benefits of Autophagy

Although autophagy presents multiple benefits, there are two major benefits of this process:

Autophagy eliminates waste cells, misfolded proteins, and pathogens from your body. Autophagy is instrumental in ridding the body of all waste that is making you sick and contributing to inefficient functioning. It removes the pathogens that live inside your body, thriving on your energy and making you experience good health. The presence of wasted cells and misfolded proteins often clutter your body. Autophagy comes in to recycle and clean them up, giving your body new cells while also releasing energy that your body can use when there's an extreme shortage.

Autophagy helps to improve muscle performance. When you exercise, the stress on your cells causes energy to go up, making parts get worn out faster. Autophagy, therefore, helps in removing the damage and keeping the energy needs in check.

Autophagy helps in the prevention of neurodegenerative disorders. Most of the neurodegenerative disorders are a result of damaged proteins forming around neurons. Thus, autophagy offers protection by eliminating these proteins. In particular, autophagy will help clear proteins associated with Alzheimer's, Parkinson's, and Huntington's diseases.

Autophagy enhances metabolic efficiency. Autophagy can be activated to help in improving the work of mitochondria the smallest part of the cell. This makes the cells work efficiently hence becoming more efficient.

Autophagy slows down the progression of certain diseases. Diseases too need energy for them to spread in the body. Thus, by starving them of energy, they're unable to function. For instance, cancer cells usually function like the normal body cells thriving on glucose obtained through food. When you go on a fast and deprive the body of this energy, the progression of cancer stops dramatically since they can't rely on fat energy to spread. In the same way, when you live on a fat diet, your body will begin burning fat hence literally starving cancer. This also applies to other chronic inflammations that flourish in your body silently because of the availability of energy that will begin to go when you're on extended fasts.

Autophagy helps fight against infectious diseases. Autophagy removes toxins that cause infections in addition to helping your body improve the way your body responds to infections. Most importantly, viruses and intracellular bacteria can be removed by autophagy.

Common Misconceptions About Autophagy

Intermittent fasting has become popular over the years, effectively shifting the spotlight on autophagy. As a result, many people have come up with speculations and assumptions about autophagy that are untrue. Here are some of the false beliefs about people hold autophagy:

You can trigger autophagy with a 24-hour fast. Neither will a 16-hour or 24-hour fast trigger autophagy. This is because this is such a short time frame. Instead, if you want to trigger autophagy within a short time, then high-intensity exercise is recommended. The reason autophagy can't happen after a 24-hour fast is simple. Fasting doesn't happen soon after your last meal because then your body has to digest the food and draw energy from it. Thus, after your last fast, the body will be in a postabsorptive state of metabolism for a couple of hours. Remember, it takes more time to digest certain foods. Foods like fibers, vegetables, fat, and protein don't digest that easy. Because of this, the body will not be getting into the fasted state until after a period of 5 to 6 hours of going without food. The reason is simple. Before that, you're still in a fed state as your body thrives on the calories you've consumed. For example, if you had your last meal at 7pm, it will not be until midnight when you actually begin the actual physiological fast. Therefore, while you'll claim to be going on a 16- to 20-hour fast, in reality, you've spent about 12 hours fasting. This is such a short time to trigger autophagy. Even then, your fast is not in vain because you'll still experience the other benefits of intermittent fasting that include; low inflammation levels, reduced insulin levels, and fat burning.

More is better. You need a minimum of three days fasting to experience autophagy. That is by the time you're getting to your third day of fasting; you'll enjoy benefits of autophagy and fasting as this will energize your body to fight off tumors, cancer cells as well as boost the production of stem cells. Even then, prolonged autophagy is not the best. If anything, it can have side effects that include providing ample ground for the production of bacteria and Brucella. Extended autophagy may also see the resilience of tumor cells because they're strengthened, thus becoming more resistant to treatment. The essential autophagy gene ATG6/BECN1 that encodes Beclin 1 protein and is vital in reducing cancer cells may instead feed the cancer cells, thus giving them the strength they need to survive. Finally, there's a risk of muscle wasting and sarcopenia that affects longevity. Although you can't dispute the fact that autophagy is incredible, you need to be aware that it's not good to always be in this state. Otherwise, you'll end up with unwanted repercussions as well as health hazards. Thus, it's best to induce autophagy intermittently; don't make it a constant process.

Autophagy means starvation. Some people believe that autophagy will make you starve. This is untrue. Although you have to avoid eating for an extended period to achieve autophagy, this is totally different from starvation. Staying away from food for a couple of days will not make you starve because people who are starving don't even have the energy to go about their lives and daily activities like someone who is practicing intermittent fasting will. Intermittent fasting doesn't deprive your body of energy since the body stores unused energy as fats that it resorts to whenever there's scarcity. This is not only in overweight and obese people but also those with a lean mass.

Additionally, autophagy breaks down misfolded proteins and old cells that serve as additional sources of energy when you are not feasting. Thus, your body turns to other body components for energy. After a couple of days of fasting, you get to experience ketosis where your normal metabolism is suspended due to the absence of new food consumption. Thus, the body begins to use ketones and stored fats to draw energy for the muscle and brain. You eventually get to improve your lifespan through basal autophagy.

Autophagy makes you build muscle. This is an outright lie because you need calories to build muscles. Therefore, building muscles during autophagy will be close to impossible since there's no additional source of energy when you're staying away from food. Moreover, proteins are essential to muscle building are it requires a vital process that is referred to as protein synthesis. Intermittent fasting limits your protein intake is limited; thus, your body easily switches to a catabolic state where it breaks down as opposed to an anabolic state where it grows. Remember, autophagy can still breakdown old protein floating around your body cells that are central to muscle protein synthesis. However, experts point to the fact that with proper meal choice, you can maintain your muscle mass during intermittent fasting.

Coffee hinders autophagy. Taking coffee doesn't have any impact on your body's ability to achieve autophagy. In fact, taking coffee is good for inducing autophagy and ketosis because coffee contains polyphenols, that is a compound that promotes autophagy. Thus, coffee supports the process of autophagy. Caffeine also contributes to the body enjoying lipolysis that burns fat while reducing insulin, thus improving ketones and boosting AMPK. Although it doesn't hinder autophagy, you shouldn't take your coffee with sugar, sweeteners or even cream as these can increase the insulin level, thus stopping any benefit, you'd get from fasting.

When you exercise, you stop autophagy. Exercising is among the proven ways of inducing autophagy. Simply put, activity triggers autophagy. Resistance training is an excellent way of increasing mTOR signaling. While exercising will not activate mTOR in the same manner that eating does, exercise will translocate mTOR complex near the cellular membrane, preparing it for action as soon as you begin eating. By working out, you become more sensitive to activating mTOR; this will trigger more growth after working out. In addition, you also get to activate autophagy with in-depth resistance training that can help in reducing the breakdown and destruction of muscles by regulating the IGF-1 as well as its receptors. Apart from fasting, the other best approach to increasing autophagy is working out. Ultimately, you can combine both in order to attain the best results.

Eating fruits will not stop autophagy. Most of the fruits are laden with fructose that is digested by the liver before being stored as liver glycogen. When you have excess levels of fructose, it's converted to triglycerides. Thus, eating fruits will definitely work against ketosis and autophagy as it promotes liver glycogen storage. The content of glycogen in the liver makes sure that there's a balance between the mTOR and AMPK. When you consume fruits with a regulated amount of fats and protein may help in remaining in a catabolic state of breaking down molecules. Even then, the chance of experiencing autophagy is quite slim.

Most of the autophagy research has been done on yeast and rats. Genetic screening studies have found at least 32 different autophagy-related genes. Research continues to show the importance of autophagic processes as a response to stress and starvation. As you may know, insulin is the hormone that is responsible for letting glucose in the blood to enter the cells, thus energizing them for proper functioning. Thus, the more glucose you ingest, the more likely it will be stored in the blood effectively raising your insulin levels and blood sugar. Even then, the insulin will only get active and begins working if magic when its level decreases, thereby regulating your blood level. It's important to understand that fasting for extended periods is not easy; hence, you'll do well to start with intermittent fasting, which, when done on a regular basis produces the benefits of autophagy.

Chapter 8: The Seven Types of Intermittent Fasting Diets

Intermittent fasting is about changing your pattern of eating. You can choose to abstain from eating partially or entirely for a specified period before you can begin eating again. As such, there are many different methods of fasting. These methods vary in terms of the number of days, hours, and calorie allowances. With intermittent fasting, every person's lifestyle and experience is unique; hence, different styles will suit different people. Here are 7 common types of intermittent fasting diets:

The 12:12 Diet

With this diet, you need to adhere to a 12-hour fasting window and a subsequent 12-hour feeding window every day. This means that if you eat dinner at 9 p.m., you won't have breakfast until 9 a.m. the following morning. This intermittent fasting protocol is perhaps the easiest to follow. This plan is particularly good for beginners because of the relatively small fasting window. You can also opt to incorporate sleep in the fasting window, which means you'll be asleep for most of the fasting window. Apart from helping you lose fat and weight, this plan offers numerous benefits. First, it helps you break from the habit of binge eating or snacking at midnight mindlessly. Secondly, it helps in clearing inflammation as well as getting rid of damaged cells, thereby preventing cancer while also promoting healthy gut microbes. Fasting at night stimulates cell regeneration that has a positive effect on cancer, dementia, heart attacks, and dementia.

When you go for the 12:12 fasting plan, caution must be taken when choosing food so that you only take low-fat food with high protein and low carbohydrates. Most importantly, stay away from processed food. When followed to the latter, the 12:12 plan yields incredible results that include improved brain health, reduced inflammation, enhanced detoxification, and weight loss. To incorporate the 12:12 plan in your day, make sure that you leave 12 hours between your evening and morning meal. You can, however, take water and unsweetened tea.

16:8 Intermittent Fasting Plan

The 16:8 intermittent fasting plan limits your consumption of foods and beverages containing calories to 8 hours a day while abstaining from eating for the remainder of the 16 hours. You can repeat this cycle frequently from once to twice a day or even make it your daily routine depending on what you prefer. This plan is common among those looking to burn fat and lose weight. There are no strict regulations and rules, making it easy to follow and see the result with so little effort. It's also flexible and less restrictive hence can fit into just about any lifestyle. Apart from weight loss, the 16:8 will also help to improve blood sugar control, enhanced longevity, and boost brain function.

Getting Started With 16:8

The 16:8 plan is safe, simple, and sustainable. To begin, you need to pick an appropriate eating window within which you limit your food intake. Most people prefer eating between noon and 8 p.m. so that they skip breakfast. You may also have your eating window between 9 a.m. and 5 p.m. allowing you plenty of time for healthy breakfast, a normal lunch and a light dinner or snack. Since everyone is different, you can experiment with different timings and see what works for your lifestyle and schedule. Regardless of what you choose to eat, make sure you space out to have several small meals and snacks throughout the day. This is important in stabilizing your blood sugar levels and keeping hunger under control. To maximize the potential of health benefits, make sure you're only consuming nutritious whole beverages and foods during your eating.

Having nutrient-rich foods helps in rounding out your diet so that you reap the rewards of this eating plan. While at it, make sure you're drinking calorie-free beverages such as water and unsweetened coffee and tea to keep your appetite in check. The 16:8 plan is easy to follow since it cuts down the time you spend preparing food and cooking every week. Some of the benefits associated with this plan include improved blood sugar control, increased weight loss, and enhanced longevity. On the flipside, this plan also has drawbacks. Restricting your food consumption to eight hours can cause you to eat more during the eating window in a bid to make up for the time spent fasting. This can lead to weight gain, development of unhealthy eating habits, and digestive weight gain. You may also experience some short-term negative side effects like weakness, fatigue, and hunger when starting out. Some research findings suggest that intermittent fasting affects women differently and could interfere with reproduction and fertility. Therefore, make sure you consult your doctor before you start.

5:2 Intermittent Fasting Plan

The 5:2 intermittent fasting plan is also referred to as The Fast Diet. This plan, which was popularized by British journalist Michael Mosley, lets you have five days of normal eating and two days of restricted calories to a quarter of your daily needs, usually 500-600 per day. The plan doesn't spell out the specific days you should eat or fast. You're at liberty to make this decision. For instance, you can decide to fast on Mondays and Thursdays where you eat two to three small meals and eat normally for the rest of the days. Even then, you need to know that eating normally doesn't imply eating anything, including junk or even binge eating because then you won't lose weight but instead gain.

A study on the 5:2 diet found that this diet has the potential of causing weight loss that is similar to regular restriction of calories. This plan was also effective in the reduction of insulin levels as well as improving insulin sensitivity.

The 5:2 plan can be effective when done in the right manner because it lets you consume fewer calories. Thus, you shouldn't compensate for the fasting days by eating more than you'd normally eat when you're not fasting. There's no rule on when and what you should eat on the days when you're fasting. One of the side effects you'll experience at that beginning of this program is extreme episodes of hunger accompanied by feelings of weakness and sluggish. However, this tends to fade with time, especially when you're busy with other things. Eventually, they find it easier to fast. Should you notice that you're repeatedly feeling unwell or faint, be sure to talk to your doctor. The 5:2 plan, just like any other plan is not suitable for everyone. Some of the people who should avoid this plan include people who experience drops in blood sugar levels, people with an eating disorder, and people who are malnourished and underweight with known nutrient deficiencies.

Alternate Day Intermittent Fasting

With this plan, you fast on one day and eat the next day. This means that you're restricting what you'll be eating half the time. When you're fasting, you can drink calorie-free beverages like unsweetened tea, coffee, and water. Studies on alternate day fasting reveal that you can lose 3-8% of your body weight between 2 and 12 weeks. You can also consider modified alternate fasting that lets you have 500 calories on fasting days and is more tolerable because of the decreased amounts of hunger hormones and an increase in the satiety hormones. Alternate day fasting will not only help you to lose weight but also help in lowering insulin levels in type 2 diabetes patients. Type 2 diabetes makes up 90-95% of diabetes cases in the US.

Moreover, more than two-thirds of Americans are considered to be pre-diabetic, which means they've higher blood sugar levels that can't be categorized as diabetes. Restricting calories and losing weight is an effective means of improving or reversing the symptoms of type 2 diabetes. Alternate day fasting also contributes to mild reductions in risk factors for type 2 diabetes in obese and overweight individuals.

Most importantly, alternate day fasting is especially effective in reducing insulin resistance and lowering insulin levels with a minor effect on blood sugar control. Excessive insulin levels have been linked to obesity, cancer, heart disease, and other chronic diseases. Thus, insulin resistance and a dip in insulin levels can lead to a significant decline in type 2 diabetes. Evidence suggests that alternate day fasting is a great option for weight loss and reducing risk factors for heart disease. Other common health benefits of alternate day fasting are:

- Decreased blood triglycerides

- Lower LDL cholesterol concentration

- Decreased blood pressure

- Reduced waist circumference

- Increased number of large LDL particles and reduction in dangerous small, dense LDL particles.

One of the common effects of alternate day fasting is its ability to stimulate autophagy. This gives you the added advantage of having parts of old cells degraded and recycled. This process is crucial in preventing diseases like cancer, neurodegeneration, cancer, and infections. In addition, it also contributes to delaying aging as well as reducing the risk of tumors.

Warrior Fasting Diet

The warrior diet was created by Ori Hofmekler, who was a former member of the Israeli Special Forces. This intermittent fasting plan is based on the eating patterns of ancient warriors that feasted at night and ate little during the day. This plan is designed to improve the way we feel, eat, look, and perform by stressing the body through reduced consumption of food hence triggering survival instincts. According to Ori Hofmekler, this diet is not based on science but on personal observations and beliefs. When you follow this diet, you're required to under eat for at least 20 hours a day, that is considered to be the fasting period but eat as much food at night. You should aim at eating small amounts of foods such as hard-boiled eggs, dairy products, vegetables and fruits, and non-caloric fluids. You then have a four-hour feeding window. It is recommended that you stick to healthy, organic, and unprocessed food choices. Like other intermittent fasting plans, warrior fasting helps you burn fat, boost your energy levels, improve concentration/brain health, decrease inflammation, control blood sugar, and stimulate cellular repair.

Despite all these health benefits that the warrior diet promises, it also has some potential downfalls that include the following:

It's inappropriate for most people. This diet is inappropriate for most people, including expectant women, children, extreme athletes, people with diseases such as type 1 diabetes, and underweight people.

It can be difficult to stick to for some people. This is an obvious limitation of this diet because it restricts the time that you can eat substantial meals to just four hours. This can be difficult to maintain, especially if you desire to go out for lunch or breakfast.

Warrior fasting can cause disordered eating. This plan emphasizes on overeating that can be problematic for most people. However, Ori argues that you should know when you're satisfied and stop eating.

It can result in negative side effects. Some of the negative side effects that the warrior diet can potentially cause some of which can be severe include dizziness, fatigue, anxiety, low energy, insomnia, lightheadedness, constipation, fainting, hormonal imbalance, irritability and weight gain among others. Additionally, health professionals hold the opinion that this fasting plan can result in nutrients deficiency. However, you can take care of this by making sure you're eating nutrient-dense food.

Unlike other intermittent fasting plans, the warrior fasting plan has three phases:

Phase 1 - Detox. Start by under eating for 20 hours daily. You can eat anything from the clear broth, vegetable juices, hard boiled eggs, raw fruits, and vegetables. In your four-hour eating window, include whole grains, plant proteins, cooked vegetables, salads, and cheese. You can also take water, small amounts of milk, tea, and coffee throughout the day. The whole idea is to detox.

Phase 2. This week, your focus should be on high fat. Therefore, you shouldn't consume any starches or grains but instead focus on eating foods like vegetable juices, dairy, clear broth, raw fruits, hard boiled eggs lean animal protein as well as cooked vegetables.

Phase 3. This is the phase where you conclude your fat loss. Thus, it cycles between periods of high protein and high carb intake. This would mean 1-2 days of high carbs, followed by 1-2 days of high protein and low cards.

Eat Stop Eat Intermittent Fasting

The Eat stop eat intermittent fasting regimen involves fasting for 24 hours once or twice weekly. This method was made popular by Brad Pilon, a fitness expert and has been quite popular over the past few years. You fast from dinner one day to dinner the next day amounting to 24 hours of being in the fasted state. This means that if you finish dinner at 8 p.m., you don't eat anything until 8 p.m. the next day to make a full 24-hour fast. This fasting plan is not restricted to dinner alone; you can also fast from breakfast to breakfast or better still lunch to lunch and get the same end result. Like other intermittent fasting plans, you can take coffee, water, and other beverages with zero calories during the fast. However, no solid food is allowed. If your goal of doing the 24-hour weekly fast is to lose weight, make sure you're eating normally during your eating period. That is, just consume the same amount of food you'd be normally consuming without keeping the fast in mind. The challenge with this 24-hour fast is that it's fairly difficult for many people because of the length of the fasting window. Thus, you don't have to go all the way at the beginning. You can begin with 14-16 hours of fasting, increasing the duration with time. Generally, the first few hours of the fast will be easy before you become ravenously hungry. However, with discipline and taking enough fluid during the fasting duration, you can be sure to pull through. Soon, you'll get used to doing these fasts.

Spontaneous Meal Skipping

You don't have to stick to a specific intermittent fasting plan to reap the benefits. You could actually consider meal skipping. You can opt to skip meals from time to time when you're too busy to cook, or you don't feel hungry. Skipping one or two meals whenever you feel inclined basically means you're doing a spontaneous intermittent fast. It is simple; you can skip your lunch and have an early dinner. Alternatively, if you eat a large dinner, you can skip breakfast instead. Skipping meals can boost your metabolism Skipping meals is a good place to start your intermittent fasting experience, especially if the idea of going for long periods without food intimidates you. This intermittent fasting plan bursts the myth that you need to eat after every few hours; otherwise, your body will get into starvation mode or even lose muscle. The truth is that the human body is equipped very well to handle extended periods of famine, let alone having to do without a meal or two from time to time. Therefore, if there's a day you're really not hungry, you can skip breakfast so that you have healthy lunch and dinner. This fast is also convenient if you're traveling somewhere but just can't find something you can eat. You just must sure that you eat healthy foods.

Chapter 9: Cautions While Making the Transition to Intermittent Fasting

Preparation is the key to succeeding in intermittent fasting. When you prepare well, you can be sure to stay in control so that you're not feeling lost and out of place. If you want to reap the benefits of intermittent fasting quickly, you must be keen to make the right move when getting into this practice. Your body is accustomed to eating after 2-3 hours; therefore, you need to immerse yourself into fasting systematically. Although this sounds simple in principle, it's actually not easy when you start out. However, when you take caution and come up with a good plan, you'll have a smooth transition that will contribute to the success of your intermittent fasting quest. Here are some cautions you can consider while making the transition to intermittent fasting:

Transition slowly. It's okay to be ambitious about going without food for several hours. However, as you're starting out, you need to be careful not to be too ambitious by immersing yourself into intermittent fasting that requires you to fast for extended periods. It's advisable to consider starting with the simpler intermittent fasting protocols and advance to the extended protocols over time. If anything, you gained the weight you're trying to shed off after a long time, so don't expect to lose weight overnight. For instance, you can start with the 12:12 intermittent fasting protocol where you have a fasting window of 12 hours to advancing on to 16:8 that lets you fast for 16 hours and eat for 8 hours. You can even take a break after a couple of days or weeks before attempting again. The trick is to make sure that you're adding on another day every week until you're able to stick to your intermittent fasting plan. Only then can you consider trying intermittent fasting protocols that require you to fast for extended periods of between 18 and 24 hours like 5:2 or warrior depending on how comfortable you're. Don't hesitate to tailor the fasting protocol to your preference, even if it means not doing it every day.

Take your schedule into account. It's very important to keep your schedule in mind while planning for the intermittent fasting protocol that's right for you. Your choice of an intermittent fasting protocol should not be influenced by peer pressure rather, by what is suitable for you in relation to your schedule. Don't go for an extreme plan in the beginning just because your friends are doing it. If there's no way you can have your meals within an 8-hour window because your schedule is erratic, then the LeanGains 16:8 protocol is not appropriate for you. However, if you are sure you can't go for 24 hours without food, then this intermittent plan might be the most suitable for you. Ultimately, you must think about your schedule, your preferences, and if the plan will affect the other people that you live with before deciding what is best for you. This will make your transition to intermittent fasting smooth.

Don't start intermittent fasting alongside a new diet. If your goal is to lose weight and you're also interested in taking on a new diet like low-calorie diet or keto, make sure you're not starting it alongside intermittent fasting. This is because it takes time for your body to adjust to the new meals and foods included in your diet. Moreover, whether you're cutting down on meat on your vegetarian diet or you're simply reducing your carbs dramatically, it will have a huge effect on your body when combined with intermittent fasting. Therefore, to succeed with intermittent fasting, make sure that you stick to your diet for up to two weeks before adding intermittent fasting. This way, you will have a great understanding of your body, hence a smooth transition.

Eliminate snacks. Snacks refer to anything that will add empty calories to your system and cause cravings. Before beginning intermittent fasting, make sure you prepare your body to stay without food for longer periods than usual. The first step towards this is eliminating snacks. Although not evident, snacks are your biggest enemies because they're not nutritious; rather, they're only full of salt, sugar, flours, and refined oil. Thus, you must learn to avoid them in order to stay in shape. Snacks often cause your blood sugar levels to spike while loading your system with empty calories and provide very little to your gut. Make sure you eliminate snacks from your routine. You also need to avoid carbonated beverages that add empty calories and are full of sugar.

Most importantly, keep in mind that intermittent fasting is not based on restricting your calorie intake so you can consume calories within a limit that is reasonable. Rather, your calorie intake will automatically reduce since your eating windows are short. Remember, intermittent fasting is based on when you eat and not what you eat. One of the best ways to avoid processed foods is staying away from foods that are served at fast food chains, including salads that have various dressings. Instead, make it a habit to cook your own food. This will ensure you're only eating healthy food.

Stay true to your purpose. There's definitely a reason why you're getting into intermittent fasting. Staying true to this reason is the only way you'll stay grounded to the cause. Therefore, make sure you have defined the reason why you're going into fasting. This may be losing weight; fasting will reduce the level of hormones like insulin while increasing the human growth hormone and norepinephrine that make the stored body fat more accessible hence making it possible for you to burn fat and effectively lose weight. Fasting also helps in the prevention of heart disease, diabetes, as well as reduce inflammation. Most importantly, fasting will also offer protection against cancer, Alzheimer's while increasing longevity.

Face your fears. It's normal to feel nervous and even harbor doubts before beginning intermittent fasting, especially because we have been cultured to believe that breakfast is the most important meal of the day. However, you need to know that when unaddressed these worries can cause you to stop. Therefore, face them. It's important to know that breakfast is a neutral meal hence can be skipped. In fact, the reality is that skipping breakfast will not make you gain weight while eating breakfast will not rave up your metabolism. You also need to keep in mind that fasting will increase your metabolic rate and help you lose weight while retaining more muscle.

Begin with 3 meals. Intermittent fasting is all about a total lifestyle change. Therefore, you need to start by taking three meals. This may be surprising, and you may be wondering whether the fact that you're already skipping a meal means you are doing intermittent fasting. Well, the answer is no. Here's why; while you don't have time to consume three meals on any given day, you somewhat take improper meals in the course of the day. This kind of munching counts for intermittent fasting. Thus, we must consider starting off with a balanced breakfast, eat moderate lunch, and finish with a light dinner. When you get to a point where you're able to sustain without difficulty with the three meals you'll be ready to move on to intermittent fasting.

Be consistent with your intermittent fasting protocol. It's likely that you will be excited to make a change and transition to the next intermittent fasting protocol after some time. This is especially the case when you begin seeing results. Even then, you must remember that intermittent fasting mustn't be rushed. Make sure you stay on a single fasting protocol for at least two weeks before moving on to the next. Keep in mind that each of the intermittent fasting protocols presents its own unique results and advantages. Only when you get comfortable should you consider moving on to the next one.

No fasting protocol is superior. It's a common misconception that you can only get better results when you go for the tougher regimen. While there's some degree of truth in this belief, it's important to focus on individual capacity. Everyone has their unique capabilities, thus imitating someone else is utterly meaningless. Some people may post impressive results with a 12-hour fasting protocol while for others, it will take another protocol to experience similar results. So don't go for the toughest protocol but instead find a protocol that suits you.

Focus on eating healthy eating. One of the things that you're likely to ignore when starting intermittent fasting is the quality of food you're eating. Although your fast will generally involve cutting down on the number of calories you're consuming, it's equally important to be deliberate about your food choices. More specifically, focus on healthy eating, especially if you're aiming to make this a lifestyle. While you can eat unhealthy food while doing intermittent fasting, eating healthy foods contribute towards living a long and healthy life. Therefore, be sure to include fruits, nuts, vegetables, healthy fats, and lean proteins in your diet.

Know when to quit. It is important that you're flexible and adapts to your changing needs. For instance, if your plan is to fast for 16 hours, but you begin feeling tired, you might as well shorten your day. You may also be working out, but you generally feel you don't have enough energy, this is also a reason to break your fast early. You shouldn't aim to be perfect at the expense of your wellbeing. If you begin feeling sick during your fasting window, it's also a good reason to cut short your fasting and pay attention to you your health. It's better to be consistent than to be perfect.

Keep it simple. Unlike many other diets that are designed to help in losing weight, intermittent fasting doesn't require you to deviate from your usual meals to some sophisticated menus. Therefore, aim at eating your usual meals during your eating window. However, you can also consider combining your intermittent fasting regimen with a low carb-high fat diet comprising real whole foods.

Get enough rest. Fasting, by itself, is not enough if you want to embrace a healthy lifestyle. Make sure you're also getting enough sleep. Your body requires sleep to be able to carry out some of the important functions. Therefore, don't work at night unless it's important. We aren't wired as other nocturnal beings; thus, we need to follow through our circadian rhythm. When you get sound sleep at night, no doubt your body will be able to fight off the weight in a better way even as your stress and cholesterol levels improve. If anything, intermittent fasting puts emphasis on giving the body adequate sleep. Make sure you plan your day so that you free up some time for good sleep. Most importantly, make sure you rest more when you fast for extended periods.

Practice perseverance. It's unfortunate that most people that have a problem with their weight are also impatient. This is probably because they're already under pressure to lose weight, yet it's just not happening. Moreover, most people trying to lose weight have already tried other ways of shedding off excess fat unsuccessfully and are looking for quick results. Unfortunately, intermittent fasting is not an overnight success. It takes time and consistency before you can see the results. You must be ready to see the change happen after a while since you're correcting problems/weight that has accumulated over the years. Don't lose hope in the process because by quitting, you can't tell whether you had made any progress. You can stall hunger by laughing, running, or talking to friends or engage in activities that stall hunger.

Hydrate during fasting. It's extremely important always to make sure you're drinking up enough during intermittent fasting. Yet it's common to find beginners thinking that they should not actually consume anything during the fasting window. This is wrong because intermittent fasting allows you to take water, tea, or coffee as long as you don't use any cream, milk, or sugar. Staying hydrated is important in extending your feeling of satiety; thus drinking water will help you to get rid of that feeling of hunger.

Manage your fasting time properly. It's a common thing for people to mismanage time during the fasting window just as is with our normal schedules. You need to know that not managing your fasting time well is likely to be a cause of distress. This can make your journey of losing weight painful and difficult. Stop thinking about food the entire time you're in the fasted state. This will create problems since your gut will be confused. You can manage your fasting time by staying busy while making sure that you're engaged until the last leg of your fasting window. When you're idle, it's likely that you'll only be thinking about food. Think about ways of putting off hunger. After all, our bodies have ample energy reserves that can run without food for a long time.

Don't rush the process. We all want quick results, but with intermittent fasting, you have to follow through the process. Don't attempt to make quick jumps because the body doesn't work this way. The transition process of your body is quite slow. Thus, you need to allow more time to adjust to change that comes with intermittent fasting. To succeed with each of these processes, make sure you stay at every stage for some time. This gives your body time to adjust to the changes. Remember, you're trying to change habits that are decades old, so you need to be patient to make your body adjust to the process. The other thing you must remember is that fasting is different in men and women. While a man's system is rugged and doesn't get to be affected by periods of extended fasting, fasting can affect a woman's health adversely; hence, it takes time to normalize. Hence, the need to start small and advance with time.

Have realistic expectations. It's okay to have a goal and dreams about your weight loss goals. Even then, make sure that you're grounded in reality. This is a good place to start as you're able to accept facts and avoid lots of disappointments. Having unrealistic expectations often contributes to the failure to recognize the benefits you derive from the process. For instance, if your goal is losing weight, then you must really think about the amount of time, you'll put into fasting and your overall commitment. Not taking all the relevant factors into consideration will leave you feeling frustrated and difficult to achieve the results you desire.

Determine how long you want to fast/create a routine. Since intermittent fasting is more of a pattern of eating than a diet fad, you can only get the best results when you follow it in routine. This means that you will not get the results if you're only practicing fasting in a way that is unstructured. If anything, doing intermittent fasting in an irregular manner will not yield any results; rather, it'll leave you feeling hungry. Your gut releases the hunger hormone with so much accuracy. As such, the gut is able to sense the time when you eat so that you feel gurgling in your stomach around exactly the same time the next day. This means that if you're keeping a 14-hour fast regularly, you'll notice you feel hungry hunger just about the time you need to break your fast. This means that if you don't keep a regular routine, then this will not happen. Making intermittent fasting a usual routine will help you get over the hassle of being too conscious. After a while, this would be part of your lifestyle hence easy to follow.

Don't be greedy when it's time to breaking your fast. Food is the most alluring thing you can come across when you've been deprived of it for long hours. It's actually tempting. You need to make sure that you don't get greedy when breaking your fast, rather get off the fast in a proper manner. The biggest mistake you can make is eating a lot as it can lead to various problems among them poor digestion. Your gut can be dry after long periods of fasting. Thus, stuffing it with heavy food can result in problems. When breaking your fast start with liquid food, slowly transitioning to semi-solid and finally solid foods. You also need to check the quantity of food that you eat because the brain takes time to decode the leptin signals that you're full. When the brain finally signals you're full, you'll have overeaten. This means that you need to eat slowly so that your brain has enough time to determine your satiety levels. Alternatively, stop eating when you're at 80% full after which you're unlikely to feel hungry again.

You only require a few calories during intermittent fasting because your body is running on just a few calories or no food at all for a longer period than usual. This can result in having a hangover initially. You can train your body to come with the stress that is linked to food deprivation in order to get used to staying for long without food. If you realize that you can't cope with your intermittent fasting plan, then you can consider switching to another plan. You might have chosen a plan that is not suitable for your needs or lifestyle. Don't be discouraged if one plan doesn't work. Rather, make sure you work towards finding the right fasting protocol that you'll be comfortable with while getting the results you need.

By transitioning into intermittent slowly, you're giving your body a chance to self-regulate and gradually adapt to your eating pattern that is changing. It also helps in diminishing or avoiding symptoms of early transition that include dry mouth, insomnia, and digestive changes.

Chapter 10: Common Myths About Intermittent Fasting

Before joining the intermittent fasting bandwagon, it is important to have a clear picture of what it is you're getting into and the kind of results you should expect. Like with any other programs, there are several misconceptions and myths associated with the intermittent fasting lifestyle that is as popular as the benefits. Let's debunk some of the myths about this eating pattern so that you feel more confident embarking on this weight loss and wellness strategy:

You'll definitely lose weight. While one of the primary reasons why most people take on intermittent fasting is to lose weight, the results are not guaranteed. Several factors come into play. Thus, intermittent fasting will not always lead to weight loss. This is especially true if you're fasting faithfully while at the same time throwing down pizza, candy, and burgers. Intermittent fasting works well when you're on a healthy diet. Don't treat your eating window like a cheat day and expect to see positive results.

Intermittent fasting will slow down your metabolism. There's a general fear that when you go into intermittent fasting, your metabolism slows down. This is not actually true because intermittent fasting doesn't restrict the number of calories you take. Rather, it makes you wait for a few hours before you can have your first meal. This doesn't make a difference in your metabolic rate. Instead, changes in your metabolic rate will only come about when you're not eating enough, which is not the case with intermittent fasting.

You can eat as much food during your feeding window. It's not exactly true that you can eat as much as you want during your feeding window. Here's the thing.

When you start intermittent fasting, your aim should be entering a healthier lifestyle. Unfortunately, most people only go into it to lose weight before going back to their reckless eating at the end of the fast. Experts warn that this is counterproductive to the results you've attained during your fasting window. The key to success with intermittent fasting is eating normally when you end your fast so that you don't negate the time spent fasting.

It's better to fast than snack for weight loss. Most conventional diet regimens recommend snacking in between meals. Those who opt for intermittent fasting think it should be a substitute for snacking. Ultimately, weight loss is occasioned by a constant deficit in calories. Whether those calories are consumed within a four to eight-hour window or spread throughout the day is not an issue. Instead, you should aim to do what is beneficial to your body.

Intermittent fasting for weight loss is far much better compared to other weight loss strategies. If you believe that intermittent fasting is the best strategy for your weight loss, you need to think again. It is important to keep in mind that intermittent fasting is simply about exercising caloric restriction in terms of when you take your food. If anything, there's no evidence to prove that intermittent fasting works better than the other methods and means of losing weight. It all boils down to your approach and discipline.

You can't skip breakfast. You must have heard this one even with other diets that are designed to help in weight loss. It's largely believed that breakfast if is the most important meal of the day hence must be taken even during intermittent fasting. In fact, this is part of the American tradition. Although you'll be told you need to consume a good breakfast to get fuel for the day, this is not necessarily true. If anything, it's likely that you don't have an appetite when they wake up. However, you can always listen to your body and have a small breakfast. Depending on the intermittent fasting protocol you choose, you can always have your meals at a time of day when its convenient.

Skipping breakfast makes you fat. It's believed that when you skip breakfast, you'll experience excessive hunger and cravings that lead to weight gain. While a number of studies have linked skipping breakfast to obesity, this is not the case with intermittent fasting. However, another 2014 study conducted between obese adults who skipped breakfast and those who didn't find any difference in weight. That is, there's no difference in weight loss whether you eat breakfast or not. Eating breakfast can have benefits, but it's not essential.

You can't work out when you're fasting. Contrary to popular belief that you can't work out when you're fasting, you can carry on with your work out routine when fasting. In fact, working out when fasting is a positive thing. It is believed that working out on an empty stomach, especially when it is the first thing you do in the morning is more rewarding. This is because you'll be burning stored fat instead of using up the calories from the food you just consumed. You can then eat your breakfast after working out to replenish your body.

All fasting is the same, and everyone gets the same results. There are many forms of intermittent fasting that you can follow. There's no official fasting protocol leaving the flexibility of choosing what works for you. Therefore, you can opt to fast daily while someone else fasts for on alternate days. Consequently, you can be sure that everyone will get results that are unique to them depending on the fasting protocol they're following and their goal.

Fasting makes you extremely fit and healthy. Intermittent fasting in itself is not a magic bullet to achieving health and fitness. You'll do well to combine your eating pattern with proper care and exercise. You must work to maintain health and fitness in your entire life. They should not be taken for granted. Fasting alone will not give you an ideal body overnight. Moreover, when you lose excess weight, you'll have to make sure you continue maintaining it with healthy eating habits that include regular exercise and a nutritious diet.

Intermittent fasting is productive because the body doesn't process food at night. Although it's a common misconception that your body doesn't process food at night, it's actually the reason you lose weight during intermittent fasting. Your body is wired to digest food no matter the time. However, when you allow the body a certain time, usually between 12 and 18 hours, the focus shifts to other metabolic processes like cellular repair and autophagy taking the attention from digestion. Your body will digest food even if you eat at 3a.m.

Intermittent fasting will decrease your training performance. One of the fears most people have when contemplating intermittent fasting is a decrease in training performance. This because of the possibility of having to skip or having a light pre-workout meal. The truth is that a closer look at athletes who train while in the fasted state have not experienced any hindrance to their performance due to nutrient deprivation. Moreover, it's important to keep in mind that intermittent fasting doesn't deprive the body of fluids and water.

Intermittent fasting will lead to loss of muscle mass. The fact that you've reduced the frequency of eating especially proteins doesn't mean your body is in the catabolic state as it is largely assumed. The idea that fasting reduces muscle mass is based on the idea that your body relies on a constant supply of amino acids to maintain, build, or repair muscle tissue. It is important to keep in mind that when you have a large meal of protein at your last meal prior to your 16-20 hour fast, your body is likely to be releasing the amino acids they need by the time you break the fast. It's common to have a complete meal that digests proteins slowly to the time you have your next meal. The thing is that fasting for extended periods will cause muscle loss only when you are not eating a large balanced diet during your feeding window.

Eating big meals with a lot of carbohydrates in the evening causes weight gain. Most fitness and nutrition experts will link carbs to insulin. While this is correct, there's a tendency to overgeneralize the psychological effects of insulin. The fear is that an increase in insulin, especially in the evening, will result in the conversion of nutrients to fats because insulin sensitivity is highest in the morning and lowest at night.

Fasting leads to glorified, binge eating, and bulimia disorders. This is another ridiculous claim that has been continually advanced about intermittent fasting by classifying it as disordered eating. The truth is that with intermittent fasting, the time you eat is not as important as meeting your daily macronutrient and calorie goals. What this means is that you're able to stick to your diet. Moreover, fasting presents a number of health benefits that disqualify the idea of promoting binge eating and bulimia. Besides, it's unrealistic to expect someone who is on an intermittent fasting protocol not to eat a large meal. Eating a large meal does not necessarily equal to binge eating, especially if you're staying within your nutrient needs.

Intermittent fasting has limited uses in limited populations. This myth in itself suggests that intermittent fasting is less applicable to the majority. This is not true because most of the people that have found success with intermittent fasting will attest to the fact that it's such a huge relief from having to constantly obsess about following the clock all day just to make sure that you're eating after every 3 hours. Intermittent fasting is most likely to work well with most people's routines, especially if you're working. Not many people like to have a large meal in the morning or at midday owing to the nature of their schedules.

Eating frequently will help reduce hunger. Some people, especially those that are keen on following conventional weight loss diets, believe that when you snack in between meals, you'll prevent excessive hunger and cravings. Well, knowing when to eat is far much better because you get to eat one large meal that is packed with nutrients; hence, you'll experience satiety for longer periods. If anything, there's no evidence to show that snacking will reduce hunger.

Fasting puts your body in starvation mode. A common argument against intermittent fasting is that it can activate the starvation mode. That is, failure to eat will make your body assume it's starving hence shut down metabolism and the ability to burn fat. Long term weight loss reduces the calories you burn, which can aptly be described as starvation mode. Even then, this tends to happen whenever you're trying to lose weight regardless of the method you're using. There's no evidence that this is more with intermittent fasting. Evidence points to the fact that fasting for short term can increase metabolic rate.

Intermittent fasting is not for people with diabetes. Findings of a recent study point to the fact that intermittent fasting will result in improved weight loss, fasting blood sugar, and stabilize blood sugar after dinner in group 2 diabetics. In some instances, prolonged fasting will restore your insulin sensitivity, especially in type 2 diabetes. When your insulin sensitivity is improved, your body will produce less insulin and experience less inflammation. This shows intermittent fasting is important for individuals with diabetes by reducing the risk of kidney and heart disease.

There are many myths about intermittent fasting. While some have merit, others are outrightly wrong. For most people, intermittent fasting presents real benefits. It's one of the best tools to lose weight.

Chapter 11: Common mistakes people make While Intermittent Fasting

Although it is billed as the most effective method of losing weight, you can easily have difficulty with intermittent fasting. Research has found intermittent fasting to have a 31% drop out rate. There are many mistakes people make when making a switch from your regular eating plan to intermittent fasting. This can jeopardize your expectations by influencing the results because you might not see the results everyone is raving about, resulting in giving up. Having a workable and realistic approach to intermittent fasting can be the difference between your success and failure. Here are some of the common pitfalls you're likely to be making in your intermittent fasting:

Having a wrong plan for your lifestyle. Intermittent fasting is flexible; hence, you have the liberty of selecting a plan that suits your lifestyle. You need to understand the dynamics of the different forms of intermittent fasting to make sure you choose what will work well with your lifestyle, needs, and schedule. By signing up for a plan that you can't keep up with, you're definitely setting yourself up for failure. For instance, if you're working in a full-time job, have an intense workout routine and an active family, the 5:2 plan will not be realistic instead of the 16:8 plan will be more sensible and easier to maintain because you'll have a reasonable feeding window. Therefore, take time to do your research and pick a plan that will work well for you, and you're able to stick with comfortably.

Getting into intermittent fasting too soon. One of the reasons most people give up on diets is because it presents a departure from the natural and normal way of eating. As such, you'll find it impossible to keep up with. This is often the case when you jump into intermittent fasting too fast. For instance, if you're accustomed to eating after every 2-3 hours, it's unrealistic to switch to a 24-hour fast suddenly. As a beginner, you can begin by fasting for 12 hours and have a 12-hour eating window. This comes close to your regular pattern. You can then extend your fasting window gradually until you reach your goal. It takes time to stop feeling hungry when you take on intermittent fasting. This way, you'll find better success. The secret is to be patient and see a lifestyle change

Eating too much during the eating window. Although you don't have to count calories as is typical with most diets, intermittent fasting requires discipline in terms of determining how much you should eat. While it's true that you may be too hungry from too many hours of fasting, caution must be taken so that you don't overeat during your eating window. In fact, you try not to be preoccupied with your next meal because this can lead to binge eating. Instead, consider sitting down to a larger meal that is more satisfying so that you're not completely famished when you enter your feeding window. When you do this correctly, you won't feel too hungry during the fasting window to want to eat everything.

Failure to hydrate adequately. Although your intermitted fasting plan alternates patterns of eating and fasting, you must make sure that you're taking in enough water. You actually need to have a bottle of water by your side because you're missing out on the water from veggies and fruits. Failure to stay dehydrated can results in headaches and cramps while worsening hunger pangs. You can also have tea or coffee but without sugar. You don't want to take any sweetened drink that can have an effect on your insulin levels and stimulate your appetite giving you the desire to eat. Avoid fluids that are filled with proteins since they can halt autophagy that you need to promote during fasting. If you find drinking up difficult, you can consider using an app to ensure you're sipping up in between your fasting and feasting windows.

Overlooking what you're while focusing on when you're eating. While it's true that intermittent fasting is more of time centered eating regimen with no specific rules on what you should eat, your goal should be to eat healthy, nutrient dense foods. Therefore, you should not dwell on milkshakes, French fries, and the likes in your diet as these can easily undo the gains of fasting. Shift your focus from treating yourself after hours of fasting to getting nutrient-dense foods that are nourishing. Generally, your meals should have a protein, complex carbs, fiber, and good fats. These will keep you feeling satiated and carry you through the fasting window while helping you to build muscle, feel energetic, and maintain a healthy brain.

Eating too little. While it is wrong to overeat during your feeding window, you should also not eat too little. Fasting affects the hormones that control your appetite leaving you feeling less hungry. Consequently, when you get to eat, you'll only eat a small portion of food and feel full. Even then, you need to be careful so that you don't consume too little because failure to eat enough will leave you feeling extremely hungry the next day so that you can end up feeling lethargic and unable to perform any work. Failure to eat adequate food will cannibalize your muscle mass, resulting in slowed down metabolism. Lack of metabolic muscle mass will sabotage your ability to maintain fat. Eventually, you may end up feeling the need to skip fasting or even give up on intermittent fasting altogether.

Leading a sedentary lifestyle. You may likely want to skip your workout session because you're used to having a pre-workout snack. Exercising when fasting will definitely seem foreign. Although it is advisable that you check with your doctor before exercising while intermittent fasting, it's safe to carry on with your exercise routine, albeit with some alterations. This is because your body has lots of stored energy in the form of stored fat that is used up when there's no food. Aim to keep up with your routine or consider low impact exercises like walking. For instance, if you're fasting overnight, you can exercise in the morning after which you can eat a protein-rich meal for better muscle build.

Obsessing over intermittent fasting. When your fasting, you might be inclined to decline invitations to parties or even opt out for dinner with friends. When this is the case, your intermittent fasting goal may not be sustainable. You can fix this by shifting your fasting schedule either backward or forward by a couple of hours on the days when you have a date with friends so that you can still enjoy your social life without being guilty or the fear of being left out. Remember, intermittent fasting as a lifestyle is flexible; hence, it has to fit in your special occasions.

Keto diet Cookbook

Best and easy diet to follow and maintain

Casey Black

Table of Contents

Introduction

We as human are all different, the effect of these eating systems can vary from one person to another but with several modifications to them so that they can suit you, there will only be benefits. Unfortunately, there are some individuals who should not attempt these fat loss regiments. If you have any severe health issues, it is mandatory to seek medical advice prior to beginning the new lifestyle, even if you are generally healthy, it is still advisable to consult a professional.

To clarify things even before diving right into the pool of data contained in this book, it is best to understand the difference between IF and the keto diet. IF is not a diet, but a meal planner that is designed to enhance weight loss and other health advantages, the keto diet is a diet that highly restricts carbohydrates and increases the amount of fat that you take so that you can be fuller for longer and be able to make fat your main energy source in the midst of other advantages that will be discussed later on.

The main reason why many doctors and nutritional experts give the "calories in-calories out" advice is that on paper it is simple and direct. They think that excessive calorie intake is the main cause of obesity; thus, the direct way of reversing this is consuming fewer calories. The 'eat less and move more' approach has been done for a very long time, and it simply does not work. The reason is that obesity and excessive weight gain is more of a hormonal imbalance than a calories imbalance. You will learn more about this and how the IF and the ketogenic diet can assist you in correcting this.

By reading this book, you will find a vast amount of information about IF and the ketogenic diet. You will know why and how they work so well and how they can work together to enhance your weight loss experience. You will also know about their benefits and downsides and how to be safe as you practice them.

During intermittent fasting, your body utilizes stubborn fat as it encourages metabolism that results in heat manufacture. This helps preserve muscle mass during weight loss and increases energy levels for keto dieters who want to lose weight and improve their athletic prowess. Combining the scheme of intermittent fasting and the ketogenic diet can lead to more body fat melting than individuals who follows IF but still consume junk food.

It can also increase your body structure as intermittent fasting improves human growth hormone output but at very large proportion. This hormone performs an enormous part in constructing muscles. The human growth hormone helps an individual reducing body fat concentrations and boost lean body and bone mass, according to studies conducted. Working out in a fasted state can result in metabolic adjustments in your muscle cells arising in energy fat burning. The human growth hormone also enables you to recover from injury or even difficult exercise at a quicker pace. It also decreases skin swelling.

The mixture of the two can even affect the aging process in a beneficial way. They cause the process of stem cells to rise. These are like construction blocks for the body as they can be transformed into any cell the body requires, as well as replacing ancient or harmed cells that keep you younger internally for longer. These stem cells can do wonders to old wounds, chronic pain, and much more. This can enhance your life expectaction as your general health is enhanced by balancing blood glucose, reducing swelling, and improving the free radical defense.

It can boost autophagy. This is simply cell cleaning measures. When it starts, your cells migrate through your inner components and remove any harmed or old cells and replace them with fresh ones. It's like an organ upgrade. It decreases inflammation and improves organ life.

There are no cravings, tiredness, and mood changes when exercising the ketogenic diet and intermittent fasting. This is accomplished through constantly small concentrations of blood sugar. This is because your blood sugar concentrations are not increased by fat. You will be prepared to keep small concentrations of blood sugar that can significantly assist individuals with Type 2 diabetes, even get off their drugs.

The liver transforms fat into packets of energy called ketones that are taken into the blood to offer your cells energy. These ketones destroy the ghrelin, the primary hunger hormone. High concentrations of ghrelin leave you famished while ketones decrease hormone concentrations even if your digestive tract does not contain any meals. This means you can stay without eating for a longer period of time and you won't get hungry. Undoubtedly, the ketogenic diet makes fasting much easier for you to do.

Some individuals follow the ketogenic diet integrated with intermittent fasting. This is by observing the ketogenic nutritional laws while also pursuing the trend of intermittent fasting eating. This can have many advantages, including high-fat burning levels, as both are important in using fats for energy over carbohydrates, providing you energy, reducing cholesterol in your body, controlling your blood sugar that can assist manage type 2 diabetes, helping to cope with hunger, and reducing skin inflammation.

For most individuals, combining the two is comfortable and can significantly speed up the fat burning process, making you accomplish your objectives quicker. However, one or the other can be done alone as they have many comparable advantages. Choosing an intermittent fasting unit that fits you is also essential and always makes sure you consume enough of the macro ingredients. Depending on what was in the meals, the functions can be comparatively fine for both. The job performed will be ideal when you mix both of them and will make weight loss much easier for you to do as both operate in distinct aspects but complement each other superbly.

Successful stories

1. Actor.

John Cusack, the actor, is on a completely Keto diet and the majority of his life revolves around his Keto commitment. He is always seen doing physical activities with his wife, and their children. John admits to never ever getting sick. He follows a diet plan that has proven effective as seen from his movies. He is a big believer in the keto diet and the keto lifestyle.

You look good, where did you lose weight? Shusaku, the man in the center, did a diet that was popular in 2015. The year was 2015, and it was one of the worst years that American History would witness. John -John, the football player, hated tofu and chicken. He is a huge meat eater. That was why he implemented a Keto diet. It is a long-term diet, and it is relatively simple to follow. The kind of food you are going to eat will depend on your daily activity and the activity level on the day. The diet also depends on the activity and physical condition. There are those that enter the diet when they are sick. They do it because we feel good and we are looking good.

2. President Donald Trump.

Donald Trump wanted to lose weight. He was so overweight that he needed to take surgical precautions of his heart as he had developed heart problems. He is exploring various ways to take advantage of the positive effects of the Keto diet he is on. Trump was happy with the results that he was getting from the Keto diet. His heart surgeon had no choice but to say, "it is looking good. We are seeing the pounds melting off that boy." Trump said, "I am a believer in the Keto diet."

3. Kathryn Dennis.

Kathy says she has lost 60 pounds and that she hopes to do another 26-pound weight loss in the next year. She wants to get from 240 pounds to 119 pounds.

The girlfriend of professional football player Nate Washington says she went from a size 26 to a size 4, without taking shots of insulin. She decided to do the Keto diet in order to lose weight. She wanted to do the keto diet because of the weight loss, and the other benefits that the diet has to offer.

4. George W. Bush.

George Bush is a very avid Keto supporter. He has recently joined the Keto diet program and has gotten a lot of compliments and also a lot of medical advice. He started the Keto diet after he was diagnosed with coronary artery disease. His doctor told him to do away with food that has a high-fat content like meat and eggs, He was advised to fish, fruits, and vegetables and to do away with the high carb and fat drinks. He was advised to do away with all that has a high carbohydrate content. These include sugar, sugary drinks, potatoes, rice, pasta, and bread. As a result, he began to lose weight rapidly. He does not drink any high carb or fat meal. He does not like drinking any alcohol as he only drinks small quantities of beer once in a while. He can happily say he is enjoying his life on the Keto diet.

5. Shakira

Shakira is a singer. She is from Columbia, and she has Spanish ancestry. At a certain point in her life, she gave birth to her son, Milan. She gained a lot of weight because she wanted to nurse him. She could not give up on her baby. One day, she looked into the mirror, and she did not recognize herself. She realized that she was not happy. She researched on the Internet, and she came across the Keto diet. She went through it, and she did not move from step one to step two. She was determined to do everything properly. She followed what she was told to do, and she fully embraced the Keto lifestyle. She went on a diet with high fat, protein, and low carb content. She lost weight successfully.

6. Serena Williams.

Serena Williams is a tennis player. She is very successful. She is one of the best tennis players in the world, and she is primarily using the keto diet plan. She has been using the Keto diet because of her desire to lose weight. She does not eat any good that is high in carbs; she only eats vegetables, healthy food, fish, and meat. She consumes coconut oil, coconut milk, and salad dressings. She consumes something that has a high-fat content. She only eats one serving of carbs. This is a very good development for people that are trying to lose weight, and people that are trying to improve theirs constantly. Kick-off your new year by losing weight. You do not need a better reason to do it other than your desire to look good.

Eating is good for your health, and it keeps you healthy, but when you eat high-fat foods, and high carb foods, you could develop health problems, and you could get sick. What you want is to be healthy. When you are healthy, you are happy, and you can get new opportunities to be something you have always wanted to be.

Recipes

Almond Pancakes

Preparation:4 min
cooking:6 min
servings:

Ingredients:

- ½ cup almond flower

- ½ cup cream cheese

- 4 eggs

- Cinnamon to taste

- Truvia to taste/vanilla extract

- Sides:

- 3 eggs

- Sea salt and pepper to taste

- 1 tablespoon grass-fed butter

- ¼ cup sugar free syrup

Directions:

1. Mix all ingredients in a blender until smooth

2. Spray nonstick cooking spray in a medium pan, fry remaining 3 eggs, season with salt and pepper, cook to desire doneness

3. Enjoy your pancakes (2 pancakes are enough for a meal) with butter, syrup and eggs on the side.

TIPS: if you like, add some crunchy bacon

Keto bread

Preparation: 6 min
cooking:50 min
servings: 6

Ingredients:

- 5 tablespoons of psyllium husk powder

- 1 ¼ cups almond flour

- 2 teaspoon baking powder

- 1 teaspoon sea salt

- 1 cup water

- 2 teaspoon cider vinegar

- 3 egg whites

- 2 tablespoon sesame seed if desired

Directions:

1. Preheat oven to 350 F

2. In a bowl mix all the dry ingredients

3. Bring the water to boil

4. Add vinegar and egg whites to the dry ingredients and combine well, add boiling water and mix for 30 seconds until you have the consistency of play-doh

5. Shape 6 rolls and put on the oven tray, top with sesame seeds if desired

6. Bake on lower rack for about 50-60 minutes.Serve with butter or toppings of your choice

Jarlsberg Omelet

Preparation: 6 min
cooking:10 min
servings:1

Ingredients:

- 4 medium sliced mushrooms

- 2 oz. 1 green onion

- 1 tablesppon of butter sliced

- 2 eggs

- 1 oz Jarlsberg or Swiss cheese

- 2 slices of ham

Directions:

1. Cook the mushrooms the diced ham and the green onion in half of the butter in a big non-stick pan until the mushrooms are ready. Season with salt lightly, remove and set aside.

2. Melt over medium heat the remaining butter.

3. Add the beaten eggs

4. Now put the mushroom, ham and the grated cheese, on one side of the omelet.

5. Fold the plain side of the omelet over the filling once the eggs are almost ready.

6. Turn off the heat and leave until the cheese melts.

7. Enjoy it!

Crockpot Southwestern Pork Stew

Preparation:10 min

cooking: 8 min

servings:4

Ingredients:

- 1 teaspoon of paprika

- 1 teaspoon of oregano

- 1/4 teaspoon of cinnamon

- 2 Bay leaf

- 6 oz. button mushrooms

- 1/2 Jalapeno

- 1 lb. sliced cooked pork shoulder

- 2 teaspoons Chili Powder

- 2 teaspoons cumin

- 1 teaspoon minced garlic

- 1/2 teaspoon Salt

- 1/2 teaspoon Pepper

- 1/2 Onion

- 1/2 Green Bell Pepper, chopped

- 1/2 Red Bell Pepper, chopped

- Juice from 1/2 Lime

- 2 cups bone broth

- 2 cups Chicken Broth

- 1/2 cup Strong Coffee

- 1/4 cup Tomato Paste

Directions:

1. Cut vegetables and stir fry on high heat in a pan. Once done, remove from heat.

2. Put sliced pork into the crockpot, add the mushrooms, bone broth, chicken broth, and coffee.

3. Add all the seasoning with the sauteed vegetables and stir well.

4. Cover the crockpot and cook for 4-10 hours at low temperature.

5. This recipe can be done with a cast iron boiler, the cooking time will be around 1 hour 20 minutes

Pan-Roasted Rib Eye Steak with Pan Jus

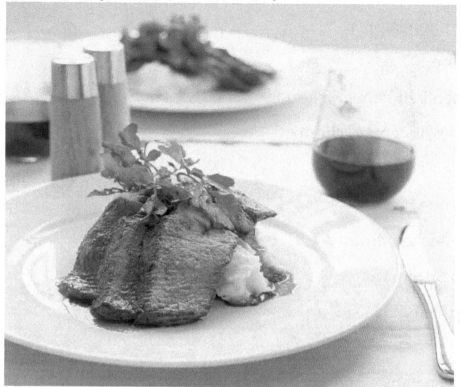

Preparation:45 min

cooking:20 min

servings: 3

Ingredients:

- 1 (1 pound) rib-eye steak

- 4 spoons of olive oil

- 1/2 cup Chicken Broth

- 3 spoons of room temperature butter

- sea salt and pepper to taste

Directions:

1. Before cooking, remove steak from the fridge for about 45 minutes, pat it dry, and salt it completely. Flip it through for about 20 minutes, remembering when flipping to pat it dry, and then again before cooking.

2. If you want to cook your steak medium or medium-well, preheat your oven to 200 ° F. Heat on the stovetop a cast-iron skillet or another pan over elevated heat.

3. Add the oil to the casserole.

4. Place the meat in the pan just before it starts smoking, then listen to the searing sound.

5. Leave it to cook for 3 to 5 minutes without shifting it.

6. Once the bottom has a pleasant brown color (you can check by lifting one edge of the steak to look at the bottom) flip over the steak and do the same on the other.

7. This will offer you a steak that is medium-rare. If you want to continue cooking, place medium-well in the oven at 200 ° F for 5 to 6 minutes and medium-well for 7 to 8 minutes.

8. Once done, put it on a cutting board for 5 minutes to rest.

9. Slice it and serve it.

10. Make the pan jus while the meat rests.

11. Transfer the pan to the stovetop, add the broth and water over medium heat, reduce the sauce by half, add the butter and stir from 2 to 4 minutes.

12. Pour the Jus over the meat and enjoy.

Conclusion

Thank you for making it through to the end of *Intermittent Fasting for Women*, let's hope it was informative and able to provide you with all of the tools you need to achieve your goals whatever they may be.

The next step is to take action that will usher you into a new level of wellness. If you still need help getting started, you are likely to get better results by evaluating your current schedule before you can select an appropriate intermittent fasting plan that is realistic, to begin with. Remember, you'll not be doing this to please anyone but for your own benefit.

Intermittent fasting is a great concept of scheduling your meal times, not just for weight loss but also living holistically because it gives you access to numerous health benefits. What's more? Unlike many weight loss diets that are restrictive, expensive, and offer minimal results, intermittent fasting is free and easy to follow through. You simply need to change your eating pattern so that you have periods of fasting followed by periods of feasting.

This book is especially a great resource that will help you through your journey in carving a new lifestyle. Remember, you don't have to change your way of living but instead embrace the new way of feeding to suit your way of living. In fact, you can still carry on with your exercise routine even though you may have to tailor it to your current situation in terms of when you eat and how intense your workout is.

What are you waiting for? Go ahead and start preparing for your intermittent fasting experience to tap into its benefits. Use the information you have acquired in this book as a springboard to prepare and transform your life.

CPSIA information can be obtained
at www.ICGtesting.com
Printed in the USA
LVHW101621070921
697193LV00005B/157